P 301 .S94 1987

voboda, Milan.

xercise physiology

Y0-BEK-428

Basic Stuff Series I

volume one

Exercise Physiology

Milan Svoboda
Portland State University
Portland, Oregon

George Rochat
Catlin Gabel School
Portland, Oregon

CARROLL COLLEGE LIBRARY

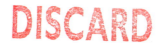
DISCARD

Corette Library — Carroll College
GV 443 .B37 v.1
Exercise ph

3 5962 00014 824

Copyright 1987

The American Alliance for
Health, Physical Education,
Recreation, and Dance
1900 Association Drive
Reston, Virginia 22091

ISBN 0-88314-357-7

A Project of the
National Association for Sport and Physical Education
An Association of the
American Alliance for Health, Physical Education,
Recreation and Dance

"BASIC STUFF" SERIES

A collection of booklets presenting the body of knowledge
in physical education and sport for practitioners and students.

BASIC STUFF SERIES

Series One **Informational Books**
Patt Dodds, Series Editor

Exercise Physiology
Kinesiology
Motor Learning
**Psycho-Social Aspects of Physical
 Education**
Humanities in Physical Education
Motor Development

Series Two **Learning Experience Books**
Norma Carr, Series Editor

The Basic Stuff in Action for Grades K-3
The Basic Stuff in Action for Grades 4-8
The Basic Stuff in Action for Grades 9-12

Editorial Committee

Elizabeth S. Bressan
University of Oregon

Norma J. Carr
SUNY, College at Cortland

Marian E. Kneer
University of Illinois, Chicago

Barbara Lockhart
University of Iowa

R. Thomas Trimble
University of Georgia

preface

The information explosion has hit physical education. Researchers are discovering new links between exercise and human physiology. Others are investigating neurological aspects of motor control. Using computer simulation and other sophisticated techniques, biomechanics researchers are finding new ways to analyze human movement. As a result of renewed interest in social, cultural, and psychological aspects of movement, a vast, highly specialized body of knowledge has emerged.

Many physical education teachers want to use and apply information particularly relevant to their teaching. It is not an easy task. The quantity of research alone would require a dawn to dusk reading schedule. The specialized nature of the research tends to make it difficult for a layperson to comprehend fully. And finally, little work has been directed toward applying the research to the more practical concerns of teachers in the field. Thus the burgeoning body of information available to researchers and academicians has had little impact on physical education programs in the field.

The Basic Stuff series is the culmination of the National Association for Sport and Physical Education efforts to confront this problem. An attempt was made to identify basic knowledge relevant to physical education programs and to present that knowledge in a useful, readable format. The series is not concerned with physical education curriculum design, but the "basic stuff" concepts are common core information pervading any physical education course of study.

The selection of knowledge for inclusion in the series was based upon its relevance to students in physical education programs. Several common student motives or purposes for participation were identified: health (feeling good), appearance (looking good), achievement (doing better), social (getting along), aesthetic (turning on), and coping with the environment (surviving). Concepts were then selected which provided information useful to students in accomplishing these purposes.

The original Basic Stuff Series I booklets were developed to provide teachers with knowledge distilled from research in six selected disciplines which have strong implications for the ways physical educators do their work. The six disciplinary areas originally included in Series I were *Exercise Physiology, Kinesiology,* movement in the *Humanities, Psychosocial Aspects* of movement, *Motor Development,* and *Motor Learning.* The purpose of Basic Stuff Series I was to take the highly specialized knowledge and information being generated by past and current researchers and structure this knowledge (in the form of basic concepts and principles) into a simplified, readable format for efficient review and utilization.

Teams of scholars, teachers, and instructional design specialists collaborated to select the basic concepts from each discipline and to present them in appropriate form and context. Selection of knowledge was based on perceived relevance to students in physical education classes at both elementary and secondary levels of schooling. Series I was not intended to be a deliberate physical education curriculum design, or to model any sort of "ideal" or "national" curriculum, but was intended to be a resource for teachers to use in revising or developing appropriate curricula for students in their school systems.

In the revised Basic Stuff Series I, the original books were carefully reviewed, each by a small panel of scholars in that discipline. Original scholar/authors were asked to do the revisions, and five of the six agreed. The sixth book was revised by another scholar. Reviewers checked content and language of the original booklets for accuracy in restating complex ideas in simpler form, and decided whether new concepts should be added or older ones deleted or revised in light of new information available at the time of revision. The scholar/authors paid close attention to reviewers' comments as they worked to bring each book up to date to include the latest information from the discipline about which the book was written. Because the original author teams for Series I identified key concepts so thoroughly, revisions for the second edition were mostly cosmetic, involving refinement of language for clarity in expressing concepts, with a few new concepts added.

The result is a new Series designed to provide teachers at all levels with the latest information from the knowledge bases underlying effective teaching and learning of motor skills. Each book, as before, is based on concepts from a single discipline and arranged in sections referring to common student purposes for participating in movement activities. Framed as answers to questions students might ask their teachers, each concept in every booklet for a discipline is organized under the student purpose where it best fits. Student purposes for moving include HEALTH (Feeling Good), APPEARANCE (Looking Good), AESTHETICS (Turning On), COPING WITH THE ENVIRONMENT (Surviving), SOCIAL INTERACTION (Getting Along With Others), and ACHIEVEMENT (Doing Better).

Teachers may refresh their knowledge of ideas from all six disciplinary areas by reading the Series I books, then referring to Series II. The Series II books identify concepts from the various disciplines in Series I and suggest practical ways to implement them in the Physical Education setting. The Series II books are grade level specific, providing active learning experiences appropriate for Grades K-3, 4-8, and 9-12.

We hope that Basic Stuff will continue to be useful to teachers who already have discovered its merits, and that other teachers will try Basic Stuff as a potentially valuable curriculum planning resource which can help us all do our jobs better.

table of contents

foreword

achievement

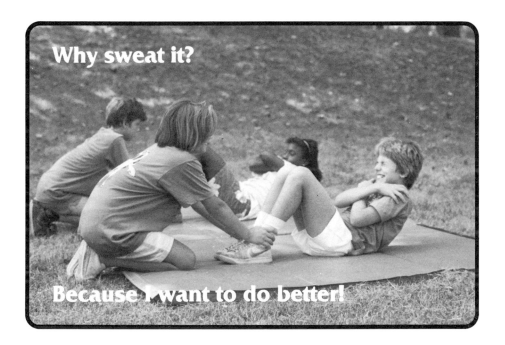

Why sweat it?

Because I want to do better!

What Do You Have To Help Me?

Everything we do throughout the day involves physical activity. We are constantly required to contract our muscles in some purposeful manner whether it be speaking, writing, or eating. Through such contractions, forces are applied to bones, causing them to move. Whenever a muscle is called on to exert a *maximal* amount of force, the *strength* of that muscle is being employed. Strength is the greatest amount of force that a muscle can exert in a single effort. Whenever a muscle contracts *submaximally* for long periods of time, its ability to continue without slowing due to fatigue depends on its *muscular endurance*.

Adequate strength and muscle endurance are necessary for satisfactory performance in any physical activity such as tennis, skiing, swimming, or gymnastics. Muscle endurance is more important than strength whenever the same movement is repeated for long periods of time such as in swimming. Strength is most important in events which involve explosive, forceful movements.

Strength and muscle
endurance training
will each help
different types of
performance

Available research concludes that proper strength training can improve the performance of events involving less complex movements of one or two limbs. Examples include vertical jump, softball or basketball throws for distance, and speed of simple arm or leg movements. Events like shotput and discus are likely to benefit from strength training because of the need to apply much *power* to the accelerated object. Strength training is likely to aid events requiring power and muscular endurance training is likely to aid events which involve endurance.

How Do I Get It?

Training for strength and muscle endurance is accomplished by using the *overload principle*. This principle states that repetitively causing a muscle group to exert large amounts of force against a resistance results in an increase in strength (and/or endurance) over time. Whether the outcome is increased strength or increased muscle endurance depends on the amount of force used in the training. Strength training requires that the individual repetitively exert near-maximal amounts of force while muscle endurance training involves working with forces which are lower than those required for strength training.

As strength (or muscle endurance) improves, the resistance required to elicit further adaptations needs to be progressively increased. The term *progressive resistance exercise* is commonly used to describe this process.

Strength and muscle
endurance training
must imitiate desired
outcomes

If strength or muscle endurance training is undertaken to improve general fitness, a comprehensive and well-balanced program which emphasizes the major muscle groups should be used. However, when the goal is to improve a specific aspect of performance, the *specificity principle* should be followed: to assure that the correct muscles are strengthened one must use training movements which are as similar as possible to those where improvement is desired. For example if a person wished to strength train for the shotput event it would be important to develop arm pushing strength in a direction similar to the angle of release in the event. At the point of release in the shotput the arm is pushing upward at approximately a 45° angle. It is of great importance to strength train at this same angle. In weight lifting this could be accomplished with use of the inclined press rather than the bench press exercise (Figure 1).

Training to improve strength and muscle endurance can be accomplished by using a variety of methods. Each will be discussed below.

Static strength training (Figure 2). Training should consist of a maximal contraction at several positions (or joint angles) in the selected muscle group. At each position the contraction should be held for 2-5 seconds followed by a 2-3 minute rest and then repeated 1-5 times. Such training can be done daily unless muscle soreness develops. Maintaining achieved strength gains requires only one training session per week.

Isotonic strength/muscle endurance training (Figure 3). Isotonic strength training should consist of 3-10 repetitions with the heaviest weight that can be correctly lifted 3-10 times. This is called a set. Three or four sets should be done each day with 5-10 minutes of recovery between sets. Three training sessions should be held each week. A maintenance program of two training sessions per week will prevent any strength gains from being lost.

Isotonic muscle endurance training also involves lifting weights. The resistance should be less than when training for strength to allow the individual to complete more than 10 repetitions before reaching the point of failure. Three sets per day, 3 days per week with 5-10 minutes of rest between sets are generally recommended.

Many exercise machines are commonly available as an alternative to lifting free weights. Strength will be effectively increased on such machines as long as the individual cannot lift the resistance more than 3-10 times per set. Similarly, muscle endurance will be increased if the resistance is lower, allowing greater than 10 repetitions before being unable to continue. Otherwise all the other training requirements mentioned for weight lifting also apply.

Another common strength/muscle endurance training technique is to use calisthenics. A calisthenic is an exercise in which the person's body weight serves as the resistance (e.g.

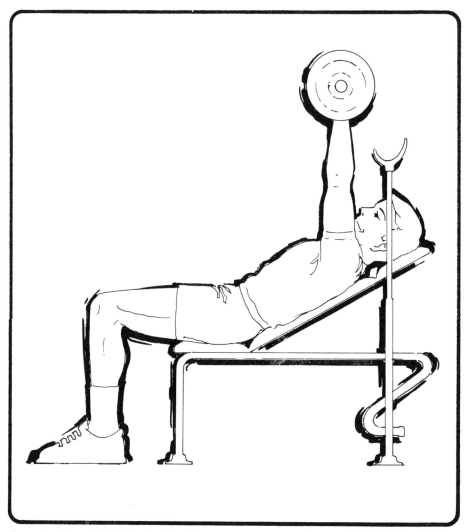

Figure 1: Strength Training for Shot Put
Training procedure closely reproduces the specific angle of release in the shot put event.

4

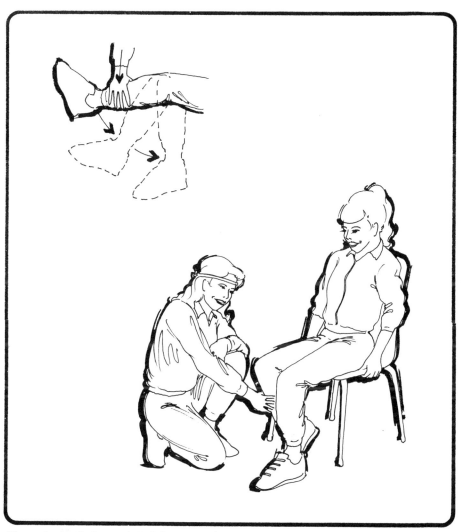

Figure 2: Static Strength Training Example
Individual performs a maximal contraction for 2-5 seconds at each of several different joint angles.

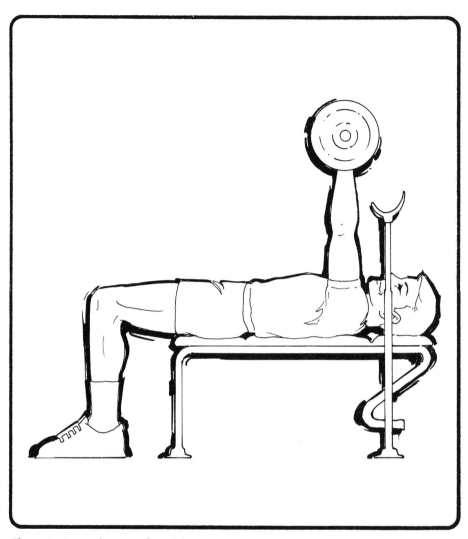

Figure 3: Dynamic Strength Training Example
Individual does 3-10 repetitions with heaviest weight that can be correctly lifted.

push-ups or squat thrusts). If body weight is so large that the individual cannot complete more than 10 repetitions of the calisthenic (e.g. pull-up for most teenagers), then the calisthenic will improve strength. If body weight is not too large in comparison to the preexisting strength (e.g. curl-ups for most teenagers), then doing the calisthenic exercise will contribute to improve strength to a small degree, but it will be more likely to increase the person's muscular endurance, particularly if the calisthenic is done until the person cannot continue.

Isokinetic strength training (Figure 4). It is recommended that such training should consist of 2-5 maximal isokinetic contractions which last 1-3 seconds each. An isokinetic contraction is one in which the speed of movement is held constant regardless of how much force the muscle applies as it moves through a complete range of motion. Approximately 2-5 minutes of rest is adequate time for recovery between repetitions of the same movement. Such training should be done 4-5 times per week. However isokinetic strength maintenance can probably be achieved with 1-2 training sessions per week. It should be noted that when training for increased strength in a movement requiring speed such as a discus throw, each isokinetic contraction should be completed as rapidly as possible.

Table 1 summarizes the important features of each of the training methods described above.

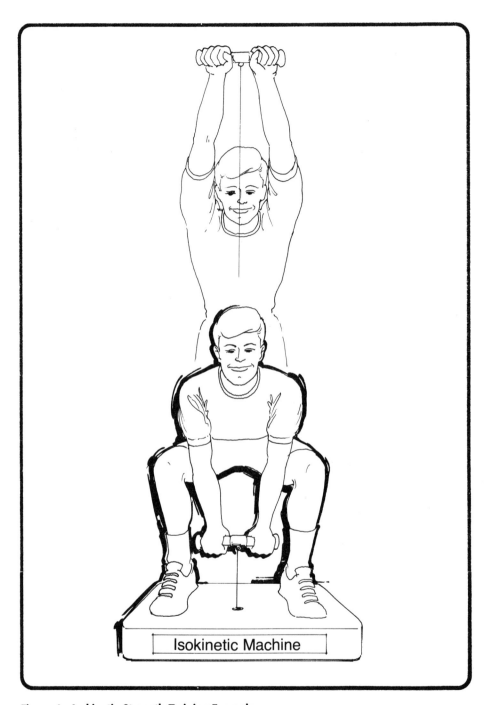

Isokinetic Machine

Figure 4: Isokinetic Strength Training Example
Isokinetic machines keep the speed of movement constant regardless of force applied while allowing the person to pull through the whole range of motion.

Table 1: Important features of the three methods of training

	Method	Repetitions	Days
Static strength training	2-5 sec max contraction at several joint angles	1-5 reps at each angle with 2-3 min rest intervals	daily
Isotonic strength training	3-10 lifts/set of heaviest weight or resistance	3-4 sets with 5-10 min rest intervals	3 days/week
Isotonic muscular endurance training	10-30 lifts/ set of moderately heavy weight/ resistance	3-4 sets with 5-10 min rest intervals	3 days/week
Isokinetic strength training	1-3 sec max isokinetic contractions	2-5 reps with 2-5 min rest intervals	4-5 days/week

Soccer can be used to illustrate how to apply strength training techniques to a particular activity. A soccer player must be able to jump high, kick a ball far, and receive the force from a flying ball with his head ("heading" the ball) without neck injury. All three types of performance will undoubtedly be improved by proper application of strength training techniques.

Jumping requires great hip and knee extension force. By doing several sets of 3-10 half squats with the appropriate heavy weights 3 times per week, the soccer player will be able to jump higher. Time spent practicing jumping will probably be of great benefit as well. As an alternative doing several sets of squat jumps with light weights on the shoulders or elsewhere on the body will be of additional benefit because of the jumping similarity (Figure 5).

Kicking involves moving the hip forward and upward (hip flexion) and knee extension. The described training for jumping develops knee extension strength. Strength required for kicking can also be improved by using weights attached to a pulley to allow for repetition of the correct movement (Figure 6).

The type of strength required for "heading" the ball is both explosive (as when directing the ball with the head) as well

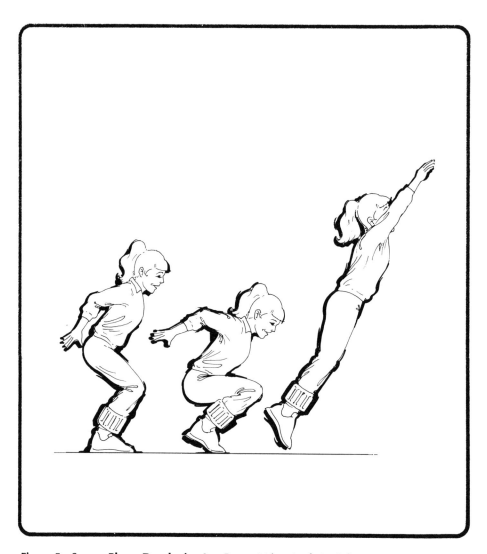

Figure 5: Soccer Player Developing Leg Power Using Angle Weights.

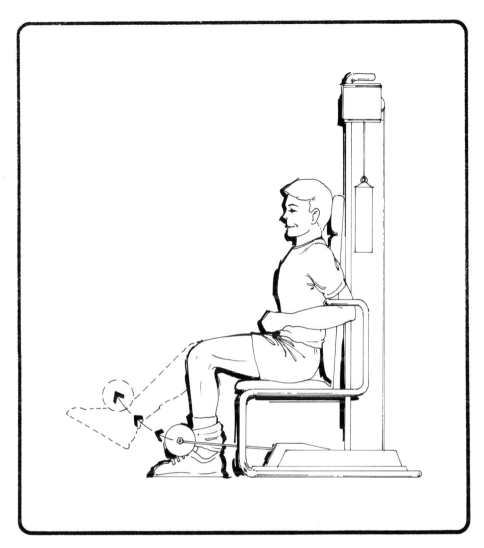

Figure 6: Training for a Soccer Kick.

as static (as when meeting a flying ball). Explosive strength training procedures involve working with weights in an appropriate pulley system. Static strength in the neck is accomplished with some form of immovable head brace against which the performer could push or pull.

Each training method has its advantages and disadvantages; decisions concerning use is of personal preference and circumstances. Regardless of the method employed an individual will experience strength gains as long as the muscles are heavily taxed. Static methods, while not requiring expensive equipment or a great time investment, suffer from the main disadvantage of not transferring strength improvements to skills requiring strength. Isotonic methods require weights or other equipment of some expense as well as 1–2 hours per training session and 3–4 training sessions per week. In addition isotonic training has been criticized as improving only the weakest points in the range of motion. Isokinetic methods are most recent and may combine the advantages of both static and isotonic training. Resistance is provided throughout the range of motion so strength improvements follow this pattern. Furthermore the time required for training appears less than for isotonic methods. Even though equipment costs are high, a few isokinetic-like devices are being manufactured at costs similar to a good set of weights.

It appears that both sexes respond similarly to strength training in terms of percent improvement, although females improve somewhat less on an absolute level. Strength and muscle endurance training is generally not recommended for preadolescent children because of the potential risk of injury to growing bones. However, persons of all ages beyond puberty can experience improvements from such training.

Strength can be measured

To know if a given exercise results in strength improvement one must know how to *measure strength*. There are three methods: *static; dynamic, isokinetic*. Static methods of measuring strength are to be used when static strength training procedures are being employed. Dynamic or isokinetic measurement procedures are appropriate for dynamic and isokinetic strength training procedures, respectively.

Static (or isometric) strength measurement (Figure 7). Using a dynamometer, static strength is measured when the individual maximally contracts a given muscle (or group) in a fixed position. Since static strength varies from one position to another even with the same muscle, care must be taken to keep the limb in the desired position and not to allow extraneous contractions from other muscles.

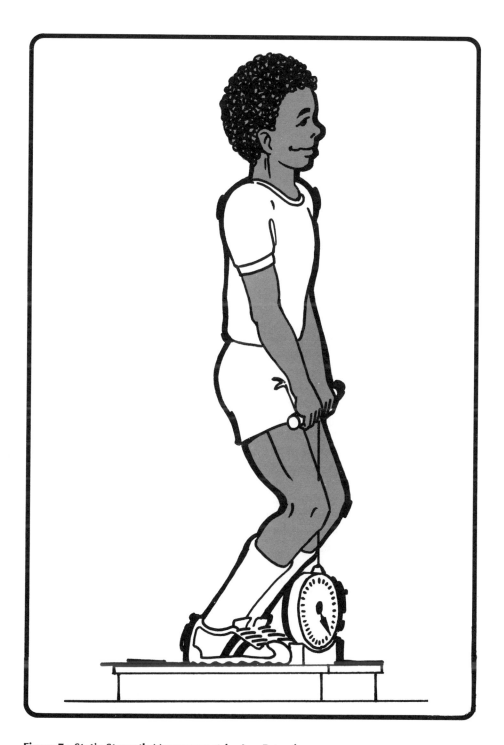

Figure 7: Static Strength Measurement for Leg Extension

Isotonic strength measurement. This is done by determining the maximum weight that can be correctly lifted only once. This weight is known as the one repetition maximum (1 RM). Care must be taken not to "cheat" by using muscle groups other than the desired ones to assist in lifting the weight or to use momentum to move past weak points in the range of motion. Free weights are usually recommended but exercise machines can serve as an alternative; if evaluating someone before and after a training program it is important to measure strength using the same equipment and same lifting techniques at all times. Similarly, when measuring strength for comparison to norms, one must use the same type of equipment that was used in developing the norms.

Isotonic measurement of muscular endurance. Using a weight which can be lifted more than 10 times, one can test for muscular endurance by determining the number of correct lifts that can be accomplished before being unable to continue. Similar testing procedures can be followed using exercise machines. An alternative is to take 50-70 percent of one's 1 RM and determine the number of correct lifts that one can do before being unable to continue.

The *AAHPERD Health Related Physical Fitness Test Manual* (AAHPERD, 1980) includes a variety of fitness tests which have some relationship to health. The sit-up test is included in this battery and is recommended as the method for assessing the strength/muscle endurance of abdominal (and hip flexor) muscles. Instructions and norms for ages 5 through 18 of both sexes are available in the test manual. The National Children and Youth Fitness Study published in *JOPERD* in January, 1985 updated and improved the norms in the test manual.

The *AAHPERD Youth Fitness Test Manual* (Hunsicker & Reiff, 1976) includes calisthenic tests of upper body strength: pull-up (boys) or flexed arm hang (girls). Instructions and norms for ages 9-17 are available in the test manual.

Isokinetic strength measurement. This requires use of special "accommodating resistance" equipment which controls the movement speed. The maximum force and power of a muscle group can be determined.

Why Does It Happen That Way?

There are two processes involved with strength improvements from training: 1) alterations in the neural mechanisms involved with muscle contraction; 2) increased force from existing units within the muscle.

The neural impulses sent from the brain to cause a muscle to contract are of two types: those which excite the muscle (excitatory impulses); those which interfere with muscular contraction (inhibitory impulses). Strength training causes a decrease in inhibitory impulses, an increase in excitatory impulses, or both. The net effect is an increase in strength due to the increase in the amount of force the muscle exerts.

Within the muscle itself existing muscle fibers also change by increasing in size. Each muscle fiber is composed of microscopically smaller fiber-like structures called filaments. The filaments slide back and forth when the muscle contracts and relaxes.

Strength training increases both the amount and the rate of build-up of protein from simpler units (amino acids) on the filament's microscopic level. The level of male sex hormone may have some influence on these processes, thereby partly accounting for the observable differences in strength between the sexes. It should be noted that social influences on females undoubtedly contribute to strength differences between the sexes. The level of male sex hormone as well as a size advantage favoring males may also account for the greater absolute increases in strength of males compared to females when exposed to similar degrees of strength training. The net effect of the build-up of protein is that each muscle fiber grows larger and stronger causing the muscle as a whole to have more strength.

Although strength is but one of many factors which determine overall performance, with greater strength the individual is likely to be able to do more forceful or powerful movements. For example, the speed of a tennis serve is likely to increase with greater strength. A shot putter may experience a similar improvement in performance with greater strength in the muscles used in the shot put. In repetitive activities, performance is likely to improve from increased muscle endurance and possibly even from enhanced strength. For example, most swimmers are not required to exert maximal amounts of force at one moment. Rather, muscles must repeatedly contract submaximally for varied periods of time. If a swimmer, through proper training, develops greater strength in the muscles required in his stroke, repeated contractions of a given sub-maximal force will be easier because the contractions will constitute a smaller percentage of the swimmer's maximal capacity. Thus after a given period of time, fatigue will lessen. As an alternative the swimmer can repeatedly exert an increasing level of submaximal force without undue fatigue, causing the swimmer to move through the water more rapidly. In either case overall performance is likely to improve.

In many instances our bodies are used strenuously for short periods of time. The class of activities is referred to as *anaerobic* and it includes all high-intensity performances lasting 1-2 minutes. Sport examples include track and swimming sprint events and some gymnastic routines. Anaerobic performances can be positively influenced by proper training.

How?

Anaerobic training must be task-specific

When training to improve anaerobic performances, activities should reproduce the movements in the actual task as closely as possible and should progressively increase in difficulty. Furthermore, as much high intensity work should be involved as can be tolerated without causing boredom or avoidance. Because such training is extremely exhausting, other types of training are often interjected into anaerobic training so that the performer is not inclined to quit.

Training for anaerobic power differs from training for anaerobic endurance

Training to improve short term anaerobic performances (e.g. sprinting) should involve intervals of maximal exercise lasting 30 seconds or less interspersed with rest pauses of 2-3 times as long as the exercise bout. After several such work/rest intervals a longer rest of 15-20 minutes is needed before another series is undertaken. The number of such series accomplished in one day depends upon performer willingness and goals. Those with higher goals are usually willing to do more work.

Anaerobic endurance training

Training to improve long term anaerobic performances should involve work intervals of between 30 seconds and about 2 minutes in length. Generally, the longer the work interval the longer the recovery period required before starting the next bout. For example, if the work intervals last 30 seconds the recovery period should last no longer than 1-2 minutes. If the work intervals last 1-2 minutes then the recovery period should last between 2-5 minutes. Again high intensity work is required. A rule of thumb is that the performer should exercise at no less than 85-90% maximum effort in each work interval. In running, for example, a good way to gauge intensity is for the performer to run practice intervals at a pace which is 85-90% of his or her best time (Table 2). The optimal number of such training sessions per week should be no fewer than three. Highly trained athletes sometimes train as much as 6 days/week.

The game of soccer illustrates how anaerobic training procedures can be used. A soccer player must be able to sprint for short distances as fast as possible. To increase his/her sprinting speed, the soccer player should run repeated 5-15 sec sprints with 10-45 sec rests between the runs. In the game the player must also run fast repeatedly without being able to fully recover. Therefore his/her training should focus on improving long term anaerobic performance as well. This can be accomplished by doing several hard runs lasting 1-2 minutes with 4-5 minutes of recovery between each run. With time the player's ability to do short and long term anaerobic performance will improve.

Anaerobic performance can be measured to determine training effect

Knowledge of how to measure anaerobic performances is necessary to detect if training is having a beneficial effect. The basic technique is for an individual to perform as rapidly as possible over a given short distance. If the distance is such that the performance lasts less than 10-15 seconds it is said to be a test of *anaerobic power*. An example would be a 50-yard dash with a running start, a 440-yard run, or a 100-yard swim.

Table 2: Method of determining training pace which requires competitor to perform at 90% of maximum effort.

Assume: Competitor's best time for quarter mile is 55 seconds:

$$\frac{\text{Distance Run}}{\text{Time}} = \frac{440 \text{ yds}}{55 \text{ sec}} = \frac{8 \text{ yds}}{\text{sec}}$$

A pace which is 90% of this time is:

$$(.9) \frac{(8 \text{ yds})}{\text{sec}} = 7.2 \text{ yds/sec}$$

Therefore: 440 yds at this pace is:

$$\frac{440 \text{ yds}}{7.2 \text{ yds/sec}} = 61.1 \text{ sec}$$

Likewise: 330 yds at this pace:

$$\frac{330 \text{ yds}}{7.2 \text{ yds/sec}} = 46.0 \text{ sec}$$

Note: Pace at any other distance is determined in a similar manner.

Why?

ATP production
provides the needed
energy for muscle
contraction

While exercising one must be able to produce energy to do the work. A muscle chemical, adenosine triphosphate (ATP), provides the needed energy for muscle contraction. The most efficient means of producing ATP for the exercising muscles is through the use of oxygen. The term aerobic refers to this form of ATP production. Oxygen must enter through the lungs and be transported by the cardiovascular system to the sites within the muscle where it is needed.

The entire process of transporting oxygen to the exercising muscles takes several minutes to reach full capacity. Since anaerobic performances last two minutes or less the muscle tissues will have an inadequate supply of oxygen. Yet ATP is still needed for muscle contraction. In this case other nonoxidative or anaerobic means of producing ATP must be relied upon. These include utilizing stores of raw ATP within muscle tissue and another product called creatine phosphate (CP). CP can easily be used to produce more ATP without the need for oxygen but the supply is limited. Finally, stored muscle glycogen, the form in which carbohydrate is stored in the muscle, can also be broken down anaerobically to produce ATP and a byproduct called lactic acid. This process is referred to as anaerobic glycolysis. Anaerobic performances are so named because of their reliance on these three nonoxidative sources of ATP.

Anaerobic
performances utilize
three non-oxidative
sources of ATP

Evidence has indicated that intense anaerobic training can increase the levels of ATP, CP, and glycogen stores within the muscle as well as improve its ability to engage in anaerobic glycolysis. Furthermore anaerobic training may result in an improved ability to tolerate lactic acid accumulation. Lactic acid is considered a major contributing factor to muscle fatigue. With a greater tolerance for lactic acid accumulation a muscle can do more exercise utilizing ATP from anaerobic glycolysis before becoming fatigued. Finally, improved anaerobic capacity may result from an improved strength of muscle tissue, enabling the trained muscle to do the same amount of anaerobic exercise by working at a lesser proportion of its capacity. The net effect of all of the above changes is that anaerobic performance improves.

What Else?

Aerobic endurance is needed for long periods of rhythmic low intensity muscle contractions

In many instances we wish to continue doing an activity for a long period of time. Examples include hiking or skiing for an entire day or playing recreational tennis for two hours. Our ability to do so depends on a large extent on our level of *aerobic endurance* (Figure 8). Virtually all activities which involve rhythmic low intensity muscle contractions for long periods rely upon aerobic endurance. Persons wishing to engage successfully in such activities will find that their performance improves with proper training.

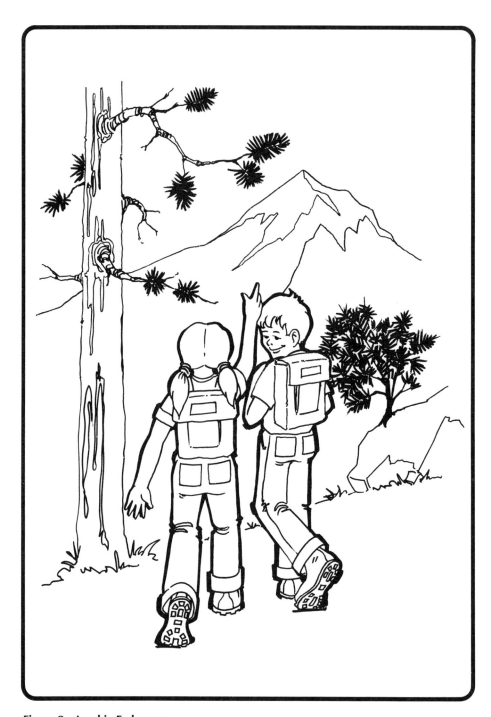

Figure 8: Aerobic Endurance
Rhythmic low intensity exercise done for long periods of time.

How?

In the position statement on fitness guidelines by the American College of Sports Medicine (ACSM, 1978), four basic elements were identified as needing consideration when training to improve aerobic endurance: mode; intensity; duration; frequency of exercise. A training program which does not contain all four to an adequate degree is not likely to be effective.

The *mode of exercise* may be any form of large muscle activity which is rhythmic. Running, swimming, cycling, cross country, and downhill skiing are all proper modes of exercise. Games like soccer, basketball, racquetball, or tennis also involve rhythmic large muscle activity. These games are also appropriate modes provided the elements of intensity, duration, and frequency are also present.

Intensity is how hard a person exercises. The simplest way to measure the intensity of exercise is for the person to monitor his or her heart rate (HR) during or immediately after exercise at the brachial or carotid arteries (Figure 9). Care should be taken not to press too hard if measuring at the carotid as this can change the rhythm of the heart. Heart rate is used to monitor exercise intensity because under most circumstances it is directly related to the amount of oxygen consumed by the individual. To measure oxygen consumption requires expensive laboratory equipment and therefore is impractical to monitor in the field.

Although everyone is different, HR generally should be between 60 and 90 percent of HR reserve; this overloads the aerobic capacity of the individual to a sufficient degree to cause it to increase. For purposes of simplicity, this is roughly equivalent to having an exercise HR between 150 and 190 beats/min for persons ages 12-19. This range is called the target HR zone. For persons starting with lower than average aerobic endurance such as those who have difficulty running more than a short distance, an exercising HR as low as 130 may still do some good while the HR may need to be raised to 190-195 to gain maximal benefit for the athlete.

A person's maximum HR slowly declines with age. Therefore the target HR zone mentioned above should slowly drop as well. Data on a desirable training intensity for children under age 12 is very limited but a reasonable estimate for the target HR zone is 155-195 beats/min for the 6-12 year old (Table 3).

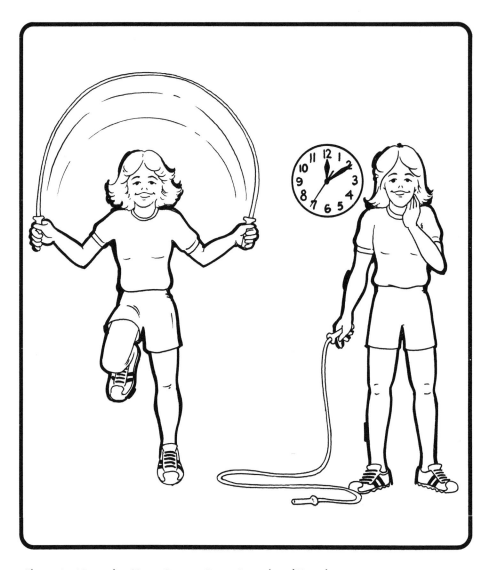

Figure 9: Measuring Heart Rate to Gauge Intensity of Exercise.

Table 3: Target HR zone for gauging exercise intensity in healthy persons.

Age Range (years)	Target HR Zone (beats/min.)
6-12	155-195 (?)
12-19	150-190
20-29	145-182
30-39	139-173
40-49	133-164
50-59	127-155
60-69	120-145

Duration is the amount of time a person exercises. The recommended range of exercise durations for developing and maintaining aerobic endurance is 15-60 minutes per day (Figure 10). This is not a recommended starting point as an unfit individual should slowly work up to such levels of exercise. Intensity and duration of exercise interact in determining a training outcome. For less fit and/or older individuals, longer durations of exercise at the lower end of the target HR zone are recommended over shorter durations at the upper end of the zone. An alternative form of training called *interval training* can also be used to improve exercise duration. In this case the individual trains for 3-5 minute intervals with rest periods of similar length between each training bout. Whether using continuous or interval training methods, the more work done the greater the improvement in aerobic endurance. Thus endurance athletes often spend several hours each day in training.

Frequency refers to how often a person exercises. The recommended frequency of aerobic exercise is 3-5 days per week. Persons who exercise in excess of 5 days per week (and also in excess of 60 minutes per day) are at higher risk of developing orthopedic injuries, particularly when running.

Training must be progressive

It must be remembered that as with any form of training, aerobic endurance training must be progressive. Unless progression occurs the training benefit derived from specific exercise levels will slowly plateau and eventually only contribute to maintaining existing fitness.

To summarize, if the mode of exercise involves large, rhythmic muscular activity at an intensity to bring the HR into

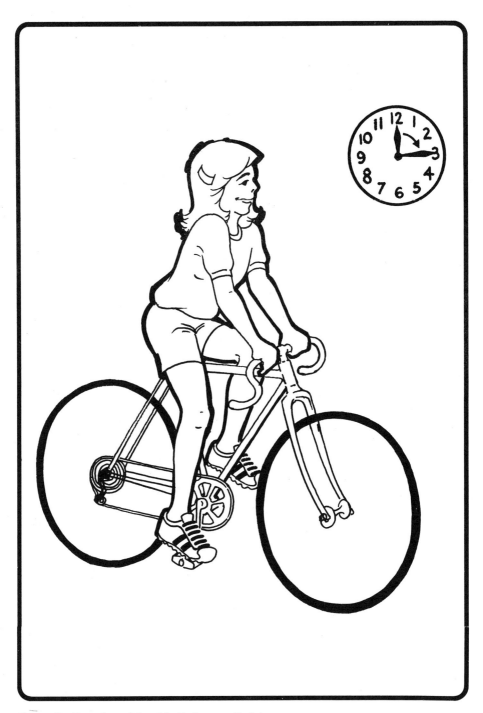

Figure 10: Duration of Aerobic Endurance Training
The recommended minimum duration of exercise is 15 minutes a day.

the appropriate zone and if that exercise is done at least 15 minutes per day and 3 days per week, the aerobic endurance capacity of most persons is likely to improve. Such training is not likely to cause an improvement if one or more of these basic elements (intensity, duration, frequency, and mode) is not present to an adequate degree.

As an example assume that a girl prefers tennis as a mode for improving her aerobic fitness. She plays tennis for ½ hour/day, 3 days/week. Periodically she measures her HR after a rally and it is 160 beats/min. Like most people she walks to pick up balls between serves and in so doing her HR drops to 115 beats/min. Because her HR was not maintained at the level of 160 beats/min throughout the half hour, she is likely to experience less benefit from the training than someone who jogs to pick up balls between points.

The soccer player requires aerobic endurance training in addition to strength and anaerobic training. A good way for the player to train would be to continuously run for several miles each day, perhaps while dribbling a ball to help make the running as similar as possible to actual playing conditions (Figure 11). As an alternative the player could run repeated 5 minute intervals with 3-5 minutes of walking between runs. Such running should be done fast enough to maintain the player's HR within the desired target HR zone. Since the player is an athlete she/he may wish to keep her/his HR near the upper end of the target HR zone and train 5-6 days per week to obtain the greatest amount of overload (Figure 12).

Aerobic endurance is tested by speed or distance in a given time frame

Being able to document the positive effect of training is vitally important from a motivational as well as physiological point of view. The simplest and best method for measuring aerobic endurance performance is by determining how fast an individual can complete a certain distance or how far he or she can go in a given time period. Typical examples of such tests require a person to run for 9 or 12 minutes. The distance covered serves as the individual's aerobic endurance score. Alternatively as is done in running competition the individual is timed while he/she covers a given distance in which case the time is the aerobic endurance score. The *Health Related Physical Fitness Test Manual* (AAHPERD, 1980) contains norms for ages 5-18 of both sexes on the one mile run, the 9-minute run, and the 1.5 mile run. Updated norms have recently been published as part of the National Children and Youth Fitness Study (*JOPERD*, January 1985). Complete descriptions of the test procedures can be found in the test manual.

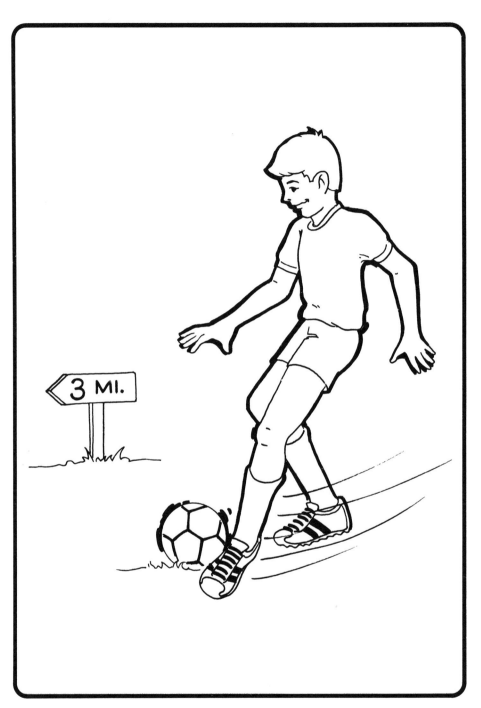

Figure 11: Continuous Running and Dribbling for Aerobic Endurance Requirements in Soccer.

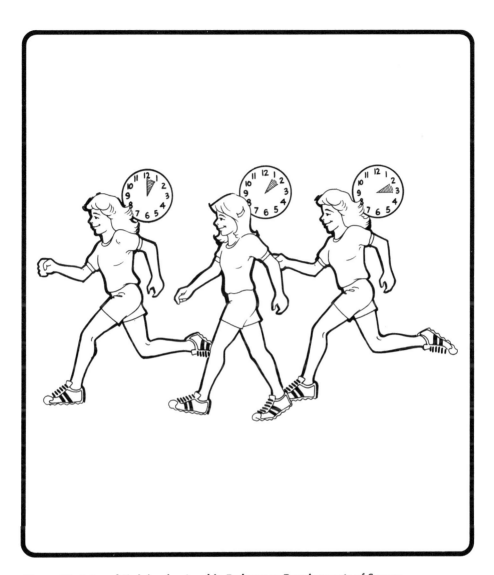

Figure 12: Interval Training for Aerobic Endurance Requirements of Soccer.

Other methods focus on physiological components of aerobic endurance performance. The simplest of these is the step test in which the individual steps up and down from a step (such as a bleacher) at a fixed cadence (Figure 13). The heart rate of the individual is then measured and used as an indication of aerobic fitness. Care must be taken to insure that the stepping is done properly and at the correct rhythms and that the heart rate is properly measured. An example of such a test has been published with norms for persons of differing fitness (Katch and McArdle, 1983).

Why?

As mentioned earlier in the text the most efficient method of producing the ATP needed by the exercising muscles requires oxygen. The term "aerobic" is used to indicate ATP production with the use of oxygen. This occurs through the chemical breakdown of two fuels: muscle glycogen (or stored carbohydrate) and fat.

Anaerobic & aerobic production of ATP

It should be recalled that aerobic endurance is a factor in performances which are of prolonged rather than short duration. Since the respiratory and circulatory systems are involved in the transport of oxygen to the exercising muscles and since these systems require a few minutes to achieve full capacity, aerobic endurance performances are ones which last longer than 2-3 minutes at the least. As a person begins to exercise, the ATP needs of the muscles are initially met anaerobically due to an inadequate oxygen supply. Gradually as the supply of oxygen to these muscles increases the source of ATP production shifts toward the aerobic means until the majority of ATP requirements are met aerobically. This interaction between anaerobic and aerobic forms of energy production is diagramed in Figure 14.

Aerobic endurance improves maximal oxygen uptake

The primary reason why training causes an improvement in aerobic endurance is due to its effect on improving the maximum oxygen uptake of the person. The maximum oxygen uptake is the largest amount of oxygen a person can consume during maximal work. In effect the larger a person's maximal oxygen uptake the greater the amount of ATP that can be produced aerobically during exercise and the more work the person can do.

The degree to which training improves a person's maximal oxygen uptake depends in part on three factors: the person's

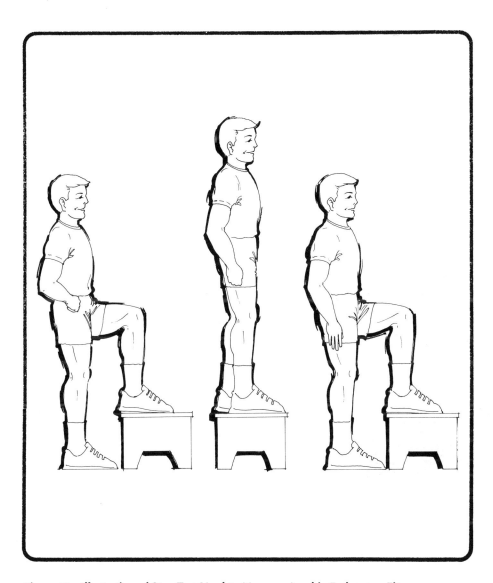

Figure 13: Illustration of Step Test Used to Measure Aerobic Endurance Fitness.

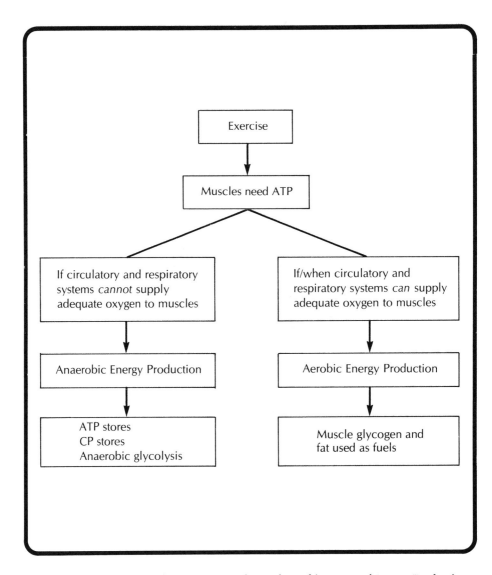

Figure 14: The Interaction between Anaerobic and Aerobic Forms of Energy Production in Different Types of Exercise.

initial state of fitness; how much training is done; the person's genetically determined potential. In general the greatest improvement in maximal oxygen uptake occurs in those who train the most and/or in those with the lowest initial state of fitness. Typical improvements in maximal oxygen uptake after 2-3 months of training range from 15-20 percent.

The improvements in maximal oxygen uptake are partly due to changes in the cardiovascular system. This improvement in the heart's ability to maximize blood circulation does not result from an increase in the number of beats per minute (max heart rate). Rather the enhancement is a result of an increase in the maximum amount of blood pumped per beat (maximum stroke volume) (Figure 15). Increased stroke volume may result from an overall increase in heart volume and/or strength of heart muscle contraction.

Another reason why training causes a person's maximal oxygen uptake to increase involves the level of oxygen extracted from the blood as it passes through the exercising muscles. Reasons for this improved ability of oxygen extraction in trained muscles is not precisely known but may arise from: 1) a greater number of capillaries being developed, allowing better diffusion of oxygen into the muscle tissue, 2) an increase in the size and number of sites within the muscle tissue (called mitochondria) where oxygen is used to produce ATP, and 3) an increase in the concentration of key enzymes involved in the production of energy from carbohydrates and fats.

Another change that occurs from enhanced training involves the body's response to light (submaximal) exercise. A trained person will breathe less air into the lungs when doing a standard amount of submaximal exercise and will remove more oxygen from that air. The total amount of oxygen consumed in such a bout of submaximal exercise does not change. Additional changes which indicate an improved efficiency of physiological response include an ability to perform a given level of submaximal exercise with a lower heart rate primarily because of a larger stroke volume. With a larger and stronger heart the individual is able to supply the blood flow needed for the exercise with fewer heart beats because each beat pumps out more blood. This is the primary reason why the trained individual also experiences a lower resting heart rate.

In submaximal exercise the amount of blood flow to the exercising muscles seems to be reduced following training. This blood flow loss does not hamper the oxygen supply to

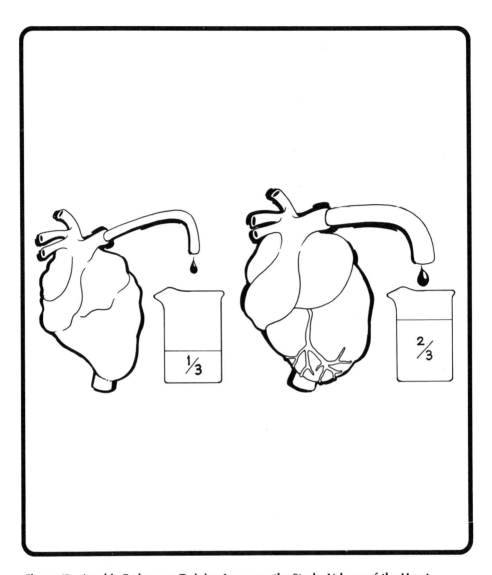

Figure 15: Aerobic Endurance Training Increases the Stroke Volume of the Heart.

the exercising muscles as they extract more oxygen from the blood than before.

Training also enables a person to respond to and recover from a given amount of exercise more quickly. There is a greater reliance on fat as a fuel for the aerobic production of energy. Trained persons also build up less lactic acid than untrained persons when doing a given amount of exercise.

In *summary,* maximum oxygen uptake improves with aerobic training because of a greater amount of blood circulated during exercise and because of a greater ability to extract oxygen out of the blood as it passes through the muscles (Figure 16).

While all these changes explain why a person's maximal oxygen uptake increases or why the person is able to perform with greater ease in submaximal exercise, there appear to be additional reasons why endurance performance improves with training. These include a greater tolerance for the discomfort experienced during endurance work, a change which appears to be psychological in origin. Furthermore the trained individual may be able to engage in work requiring a higher percentage of his maximal oxygen uptake for longer periods of time thereby improving overall performance. Better technique can also account for improvements in endurance performance.

What Else?

Flexibility is necessary for all movement

In many types of performance the ability of joints and muscles to go through a wide range of motion is desirable for normal daily activity. When this is impossible a person has poor *flexibility.* Not only does the gymnast require great flexibility but the wrestler and football player do as well. Even inactive persons who suffer from poor flexibility may find themselves limited in daily tasks.

How?

Static stretching improves flexibility

Improving one's flexibility can best be accomplished by means of static stretching. Static stretching means stretching without bobbing. One holds the final stretched position steadily for a short period of time. The optimal length of time for the stretch to be held is between 15-30 seconds according to

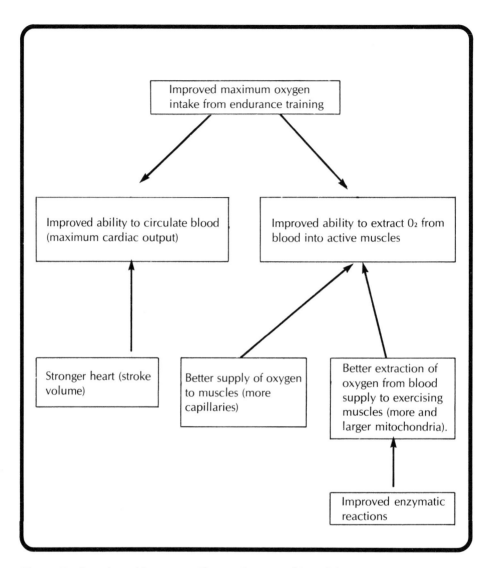

Figure 16: Overview of Important Changes from Aerobic Training.

research (Figure 17). Flexibility exercises are often incorporated into aerobic and/or strength training programs. They are usually done before and after such training. Whenever working on flexibility, care should be taken never to stretch a muscle without prior warm-up. A minimal flexibility program should be done no less than 2 times per week. The more frequent and the longer one devotes to improving flexibility the more rapid the progress. The *Health Related Physical Fitness Test Manual* (AAHPERD, 1980) includes descriptions and illustrations of common flexibility exercises.

Flexibility measurement

The flexibility of a muscle/joint is best measured with an instrument called a flexometer. Range of motion is measured by strapping the flexometer to the body part as it passes through its range of motion (Figure 18). Certain types of flexibility, such as that of the lower back and hamstring muscles, can be measured using special equipment. For example, the *Health Related Physical Fitness Test Manual* (AAHPERD, 1980) includes the "sit and reach" test. Instructions for constructing the measurement apparatus and norms for both sexes and ages 5-19 are included in the test manual. Many other practical tests of flexibility are available for measuring the range of motion of specific muscles/joints. Caution is required in following the procedures correctly to permit replication, especially if measurements are desired at a subsequent date.

Why?

Flexibility improves because muscle and/ or connective tissue lengthens

The resistance felt when stretching a muscle originates from within the muscle itself, the ligaments which bind bones together, and from the surrounding connective tissue which binds muscle fibers together into bundles. This connective tissue ultimately forms the tendon which attaches the muscle to the bone. Repeated stretching causes the muscle, tendon, and/or surrounding ligaments to lengthen and enables the individual to move through a wider range of motion than before.

What Else?

Diet affects performance

The speed of movement as well as the length of time determines the energy sources our muscles utilize. For example

35

CARROLL COLLEGE LIBRARY

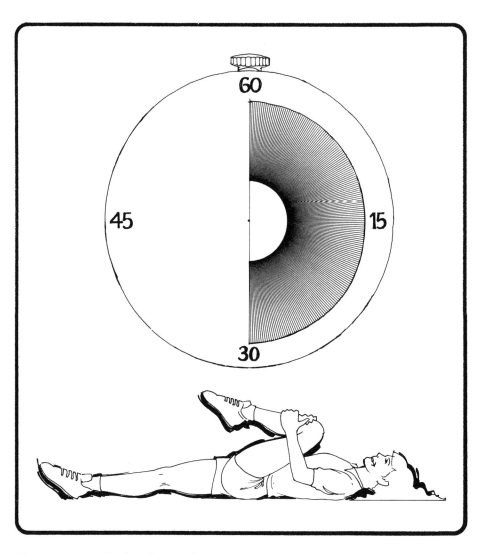

Figure 17: Example of Static Stretching Position Being Held for 30 Seconds.

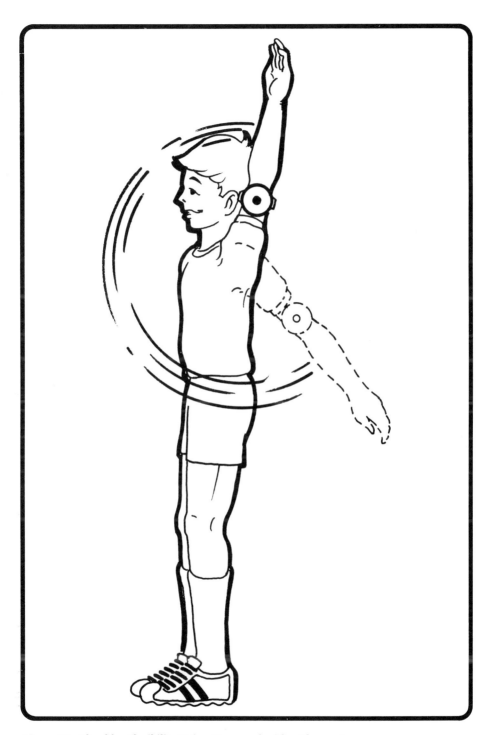

Figure 18: Shoulder Flexibility Being Measured with a Flexometer.

sprinting relies upon stored (anaerobic) forms of energy while long slow running relies on the transformation of energy from stored forms of food with the use of oxygen (aerobic). In some performances, specifically activities requiring continuous heavy exercise for approximately 40-180 minutes, the person's diet has a direct bearing on how well the person is able to perform (Figure 19). Activities requiring intermittent strenuous exercise like soccer or basketball require longer time periods before the player is limited by diet. Under certain but not all conditions an individual may profit by altering his diet.

How?

The amount of carbohydrate stored in the exercising muscles in the form of muscle glycogen is one of the primary limiting factors to maximal performances lasting between 40-180 minutes (e.g. long distance running or soccer). For persons engaging in such activities the diet during the week preceding the event can have a noticeable influence on muscle glycogen levels and hence on performance. At other times during the year modifications of a normal healthy diet have not been shown to benefit such performances. For all other less demanding activities, modifying a healthy diet has not proven to have any benefit.

Carbohydrate loading is increasing stored carbohydrates

Increasing the storage of carbohydrates in the body is called *carbohydrate loading*. Through carbohydrate loading the levels of stored muscle glycogen can be increased more than 100%. The procedure is as follows: approximately 1 week prior to the event the person should undergo a bout of heavy exercise lasting about 90 minutes which is designed to use up a substantial proportion of the existing muscle glycogen. During the week prior to the event the person's diet should be very high in carbohydrates (workouts during this entire week should be lighter than normal). The well trained athlete may not experience such dramatic increases in muscle glycogen levels. This may occur because the normal glycogen levels are already elevated due to heavy training. For such persons, the consumption of a high carbohydrate diet for several days prior to the event is sufficient.

Pre-event meal

Ingestion of small amounts of carbohydrate during prolonged exercise, particularly in liquid form as in a slightly sweet drink, will help reduce the rate at which stored carbohydrate is depleted. However, whenever trying to replace

38

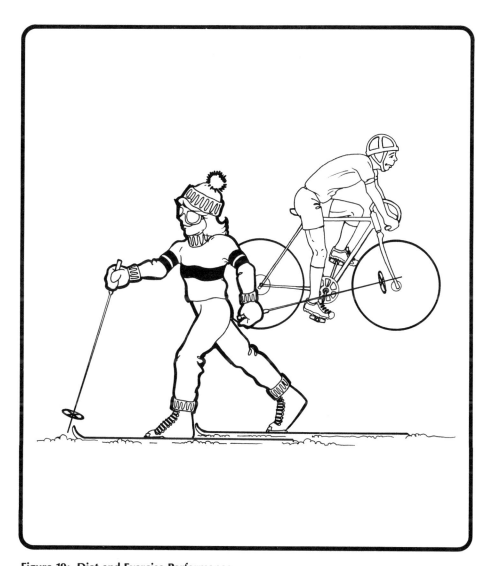

Figure 19: Diet and Exercise Performance
Only in prolonged exercise can the type of food you eat have a direct effect on your performance.

fluids in the heat, one must be cautious not to include sugar in the drink as it retards the rate at which the fluid is delivered to the intestine for absorption.

With regard to the question of what to eat on the last meal before performance, most authorities suggest that the meal should be eaten 4 hours before the event, should be light in volume, and should be composed of that which the individual normally eats. For persons engaging in events lasting longer than 40 minutes the pre-event meal should be primarily composed of carbohydrates.

Why?

As was stated earlier, only when a person engages in continuous, heavy exercise for periods between 40-180 minutes will a special diet be of help. To understand why these are the only circumstances where diet will have an impact on performance requires nutritional knowledge and an understanding of the fuels used in varying exercise forms.

Active people need more food

Persons who exercise regularly expend more energy each day thereby requiring them to consume more food. The amount of food required is related to the amount of extra energy spent. In active persons, appetite has proven to be a relatively effective control mechanism against the dangers of overeating (thus gaining fat). Of the three basic forms of food (carbohydrates, fats, and proteins) the first two are the main sources of fuel for the muscles for most forms of exercise. Protein is used to a small degree as a fuel in prolonged exercise. The main function of protein is building and rebuilding tissues, including muscle and bone.

Protein supplementation is unnecessary

A frequently asked question is whether the active person requires protein supplements to aid in the body-building processes. The evidence suggests that any added protein requirement is adequately met by including protein as part of the extra food consumed due to a higher activity status. Special protein supplements are unnecessary and often expensive. Foods such as fish, meat, poultry, and beans are good sources of protein. In fact, a well balanced vegetarian diet can supply the protein needs of the athlete very adequately. Nutritionists recommend that persons receive 1 gram of protein for each kilogram of body weight. For a person weighing 150 lbs. this would amount to 2.4 ounces of protein per day. From a nutritional standpoint any protein consumption above this amount is purely a matter of personal preference.

Research on vitamin and mineral requirements of active persons has indicated that adequate sources of vitamins and minerals are obtained in the food, provided the person eats a reasonably well-balanced diet. Research on whether vitamin and mineral supplements will enhance performance has shown no consistent evidence, suggesting that such supplemental procedures are unnecessary and expensive. In some cases excessive vitamin intake can even be harmful.

In response to the question concerning what fuels exercising muscles require to form the needed ATP, both fats and carbohydrates serve this function. The degree that each contributes varies with the severity and duration of the exercise. If exercise is light and prolonged, fat and carbohydrate stores (glycogen and glucose) both serve as fuels for the aerobic production of ATP. The longer the duration of the exercise the greater the proportion of energy derived from fat. If exercise becomes more vigorous, however, fat contributes less and less and carbohydrate stores become the predominant source of fuel. Although the level of carbohydrate storage is considerably less than the level of fat storage, there are adequate levels of glycogen in the muscle and elsewhere (primarily in the liver) to supply the carbohydrate needs for all forms of exercise less than 40 minutes. Thus in all such activities, regardless of how vigorous, fatigue or other limitations to performance are not related to an inadequate supply of carbohydrate for fuel. Only when such vigorous exercise is longer than 40 minutes do the normal levels of carbohydrate storage begin to approach depletion and hence lend themselves to being elevated via carbohydrate loading techniques. Evidence shows a close link between muscle glycogen levels and the ability to persist in exercises such as running a marathon, long distance cycling, swimming, or vigorous games as competitive soccer. Exhaustion appears to be closely related to glycogen depletion in such cases. Fat stores play an increasing role in filling the void as the body's carbohydrate stores are progressively depleted. Supplemental carbohydrate, if it is made available, will spare the use of glycogen and prolong the ability of the performer to exercise before the glycogen stores are depleted and the individual becomes exhausted.

Research indicates that the pre-event meal, when it is taken 4 hours before the event, has little positive or negative effect upon performance. This is because what is eaten usually does not alter the fuels used by the muscles under most conditions of exercise. Only in performances using the existing carbohydrate stores in the muscles (e.g., performances with heavy work lasting longer than 40 minutes) is the content of the meal likely to influence performance. In this instance the meal should consist of 80-90% carbohydrates. In all other cases the meal should be light in volume and eaten far enough in advance (4 hrs.) to have passed through the stomach and into the intestines. By so doing chances of discomfort are minimized. The content of the meal can vary and should consist of foods of personal preference. Since protein is not used as a fuel for energy production by the muscles, eating a large steak at this meal will be of no assistance to performance; it may even interfere because protein and fat are slow to digest.

What Else?

Temperature affects performance

Environmental temperature has a great impact on a person's ability to exercise. Provided the individual wears sufficient clothing to protect the hands, feet, and head, there is little danger to the person while exercising in the cold. However, the ability to do manipulative skills such as throwing and catching can become impaired in the cold. Exercising in the heat, particularly when the humidity is high, can result in an excessive buildup of body heat leading to circulatory collapse and heat exhaustion. With adequate preparation and proper precautions during exercise, such malfunctions can be avoided (Figure 20).

Well How?

Heat exhaust body fluids

In events longer than 15 minutes not only does exercise capacity seem to suffer when the environmental temperature is high but blood pressure and temperature control mechanisms can begin to malfunction, leading to heat exhaustion. This is particularly true when the humidity is high or when sweat evaporation is blocked by improper clothing. As fluids are lost the body temperature rises. Unfortunately thirst does not seem to help the person sense the degree of fluid loss and dehydration may occur. Therefore it is vitally important that body fluids be replenished to aid in sweating and to maintain body temperature at a lower level than would be the case if the person became dehydrated. This can be done by making water accessible, scheduling frequent water breaks, and encouraging performers to drink when possible. The guidelines in the *Position Statement on the Prevention of Thermal Injuries*

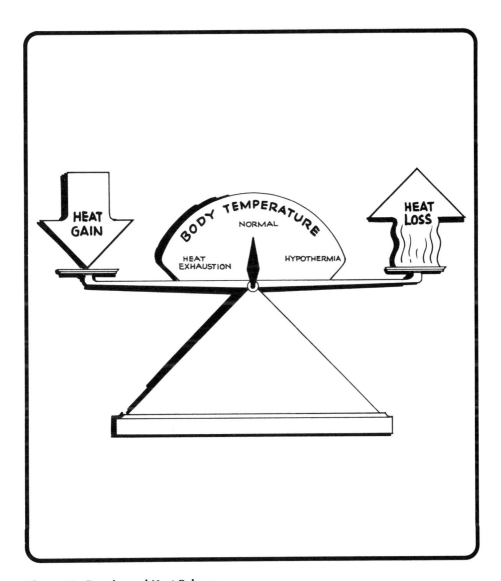

Figure 20: Exercise and Heat Balance
When the body does not maintain an equilibrium between heat gain and heat loss, hypothermia or heat exhaustion may result.

During Distance Running (ACSM, 1984) should be followed when participating in or conducting such events.

It is a common practice for wrestlers to voluntarily dehydrate themselves preceding a match in order to qualify for a lower than normal weight standard. It should be noted that rapid dehydration before weigh-in has negative influences on performance as well as on competitor health and should be avoided.

Body salt is lost through sweating

Sweating results in a loss of body salt and other electrolytes in persons who exercise and train in the heat. When this occurs repeatedly, the body's natural reaction is to restrict the loss of electrolytes in sweat. Adding extra table salt at meals can more than adequately cover any loss of sodium that does occur. Salt tablets should not be taken.

Since clothing can seriously interfere with evaporation of sweat, it should be minimized when exercising in the heat. In football, short-sleeved, netted jerseys should be used on warm days, helmets should be removed whenever possible, and all efforts should be made to aid heat elimination. Hands, feet, ears, and the head and groin regions have a particularly high rate of heat loss. On warm days clothing should not interfere with adequate air flow to these regions in particular (Figure 21). When participating on days when it is cold, care should be taken to cover these body parts.

Overheated persons who complain of dizziness, rapid pulse, and/or cool skin are suffering from heat exhaustion and should be *immediately* placed in a reclining position. All clothing should be removed and the individual(s) should be cooled by whatever means available (hose, ice water, etc.). Fluids should be given to replenish any previous fluid loss. Emergency personnel should be immediately notified.

The ability to tolerate and exercise in the heat can be dramatically increased by heat acclimatization. This can be done with a progressive exercise program in the heat or by adding extra clothing to increase insulation while training. Care should be taken to avoid heat exhaustion. Marked improvements in performance and heat tolerance can be accomplished in 1-2 weeks.

Why?

Exercise in the cold is of little danger because body heat production is increased. However, if protection from the cold is not adequate or if body parts like the hands are left exposed,

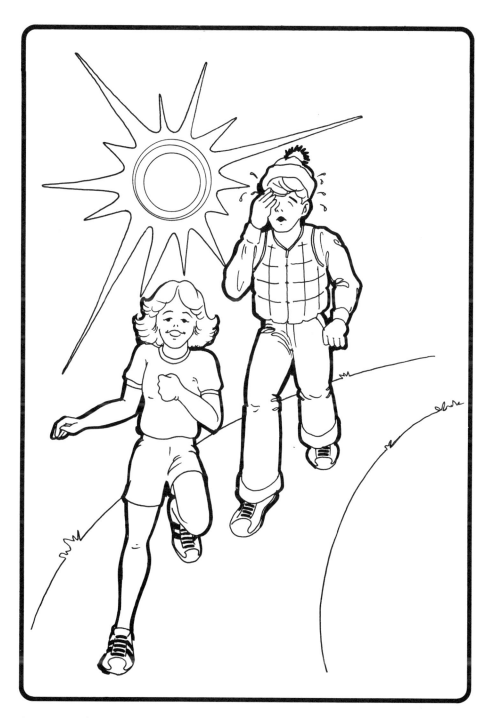

Figure 21: When Exercising it is Important to Take into Account the Environmental Conditions. The Example Shows an Over-Dressed and Properly Dressed Jogger.

the body reacts by reducing the amount of blood circulated to its surface, particularly in the extremities. In such circumstances, manipulative skills become impaired.

Persons who exercise in the heat can easily become overheated and/or dehydrated. Since exercise causes significant amounts of heat to be produced within the body, the additional influence of high environmental temperature can quickly overload the body's capacity for heat loss. Such a temperature buildup can occur even in moderate temperatures (70-80°F) if the exercise is prolonged and heavy.

Heat loss mechanisms

The primary mechanism for heat loss under such conditions involves the evaporation of sweat. Sweat is released from sweat glands beneath the skin surface. Body heat causes sweat to evaporate thereby lowering the skin temperature. Blood which has been warmed by passing through the muscles will then pass through the cooler blood vessels serving the skin tissue and lose heat. Thus via the coordinated actions of sweat evaporation and redirecting blood flow to the skin, body temperature is maintained within tolerable limits.

Why fluids are needed

However if something interferes with these processes, body temperature can easily rise to dangerously high levels impairing individual health and performance. High humidity and restrictive clothing interfere with normal evaporation processes. Since much fluid is lost due to evaporation, dehydration can easily occur unless fluids are replaced.

Mechanisms of adapting to exercise in the heat

Within 1-2 weeks of practice under hot humid conditions the body will adapt and become more efficient to the stress of such exercise. This occurs largely because the person begins to sweat more rapidly and to a much greater extent. By sweating more, evaporative cooling is increased and performance improves. The person can perform a given level of work with a lower heart rate than before the adaptation. Blood pressure during exercise is more stable and there is evidence that plasma volume increases. All these changes contribute to greater efficiency when exercising in the heat.

What Else?

Aids to performance: fact and fiction

Persons concerned with achieving maximal performance seem particularly susceptible to the testimony of popular and successful athletes and coaches regarding performance aids. Yet very few aids are likely to be beneficial to many people in light of the complexity of individual performance differences. A few aids may be beneficial to some but not others while most will have no effect or even a potentially harmful effect on the individual or his performance.

Based on current literature there is no evidence of a standard beneficial effect on performance from vitamin and mineral supplements, gelatin, oxygen inhalation before or after performance, hypnosis, amphetamines, alcohol, tobacco, or marijuana. As discussed earlier vitamin and mineral supplements are unnecessary. Use of oxygen allegedly to aid performance appears to be psychological in origin. While amphetamines cause a person to become more emotionally aroused, they have not demonstrated noticeable and reproducible effects upon performance. Amphetamines may lead to psychological dependency as well as mask symptoms of potentially lethal circulatory collapse. Since the use of such drugs has been declared illegal by sports-governing bodies, it seems undesirable to resort to amphetamines to aid performance.

Blood doping

Blood doping is a technique of withdrawing red blood cells from an individual and later injecting the same cells back into the donor. Oxygen is transported throughout the body by red blood cells. Recent evidence suggests that by artificially raising the number of red blood cells the performer is able to consume more oxygen and increase endurance. Although effective, such practices are contrary to the spirit of the anti-doping regulations of many national and international athletic organizations and should be discouraged.

Anabolic steroids

Anabolic steroids are synthetically produced substances which chemically reproduce the muscle building characteristics of male sex hormones. Many athletes (weight lifters, shot putters, discus and hammer throwers) involved in activities requiring great strength allegedly take large doses of these steroids in addition to training to accelerate the expected strength gains.

Research has not found consistent results concerning the effectiveness of such practices. For reasons of safety, the dosages which have been used in research studies are considerably below those which are ingested by athletes in the field. The American College of Sports Medicine recently revised its earlier position statement on this subject, advising against the use of steroids (ACSM, 1984). In light of the known harmful effects on blood and liver with prolonged use of anabolic steroids, and the fact that such drugs are on the banned list of many national and international athletic organizations, use of such drugs should be discouraged.

A few aids have been found to benefit performance in specific ways. The high carbohydrate diet discussed earlier prolongs endurance performance (see carbohydrate loading). Water intake is necessary and will aid endurance performances in warm temperatures (see fluid needs in the heat).

Warm-up can help maximize anaerobic performances

Warm-up, or active rehearsal prior to the event, warms the muscles. The warm-up can help maximize anaerobic performances in particular (as in sprinting). It loosens the muscles, tendons, and ligaments, making them less susceptible to injury and increases the blood flow to the heart muscle. On subsequent maximal exertion this will lead to fewer rhythm abnormalities. Significant warm-up is not likely to aid prolonged endurance performances because the increased body temperature shifts the blood flow away from the exercising muscles to the skin. In such events, prior cooling of the performer can be beneficial.

Caffeine benefits prolonged endurance performance

Finally, caffeine has been demonstrated to have a beneficial effect on prolonged endurance performance by promoting the use of fat as a fuel, thereby saving carbohydrate. As with any other substance taken to artificially increase performance, use of caffeine for such purposes should be discouraged.

Table 4: Summary of the Effects of Selected Aids to Performance

No Beneficial Effect	Variable	Beneficial Effect
Vitamin supplements	Anabolic steroids	Carbohydrate diet for prolonged endurance
Mineral supplements		Water when exercising in the heat
Gelatin		Warm up for maximal anaerobic events
O_2 inhalation		Caffeine for prolonged endurance
Hypnosis		Blood doping
Amphetamines		
Alcohol		
Tobacco		
Marijuana		

appearance

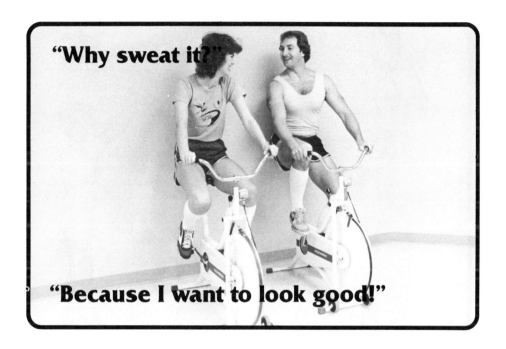

"Why sweat it?"

"Because I want to look good!"

What Do You Have To Help Me?

**Strength training
leads to increased
muscle bulk**

Males' interest in building muscles is primarily related to feeling and looking more masculine. Females sometimes wish to develop bigger muscles but more often they try to avoid becoming too muscular with exercise. Strength training can lead to increases in muscle bulk (muscle hypertrophy). Most females experience smaller bulk changes. Therefore strength training provides opportunities for both males and females to improve their appearance (Figure 22).

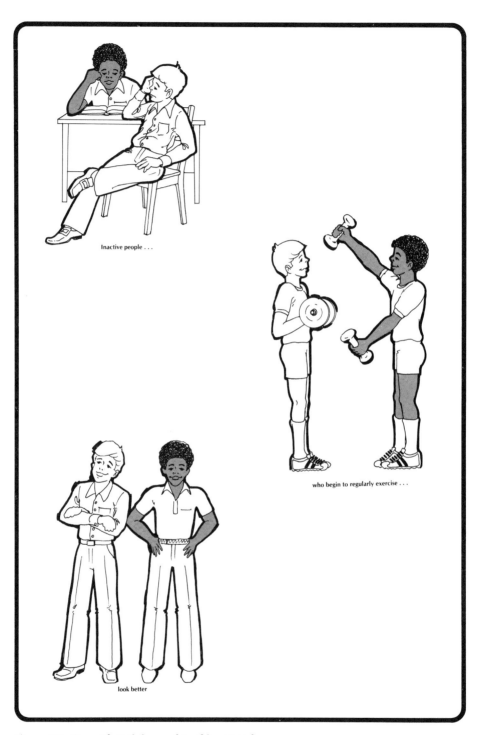

Inactive people . . .

who begin to regularly exercise . . .

look better

Figure 22: Strength Training and Looking Good

How Do I Get It?

Muscle bulk is increased by dynamic strength training

The strength training techniques discussed in Chapter 1 can lead to muscle hypertrophy. The most effective technique involves *dynamic strength training.* Sets of 10 repetitions with the heaviest weight that can be lifted correctly 10 times are usually more effective than sets of fewer repetitions with heaver weights. There are considerable individual differences in such training adaptations. As a result a trial and error approach to choosing a muscle bulking program is often used. The total amount of work a muscle is required to do in addition to the degree of difficulty affects the rate of hypertrophy. Thus the person who does 4 sets of 10 repetitions per set will likely experience more gain in muscle bulk than the person doing only one set. Any muscle building program should be designed to symmetrically develop the body in a pleasing manner rather than focus on a single region such as the upper torso (Figure 23).

Persons desiring to fill out a lanky frame often resort to high caloric, high protein diets in addition to strength training. However there is little evidence that the extra protein is used for muscle development.

Why Does It Happen That Way?

Muscle "bulk up" is related to hormones

The precise mechanisms which cause a muscle to build up bulk when strength trained are unknown but the changes have been related to an increase in size and/or number of muscle fibers. Evidence suggests that the response is related to the individual male sex hormone level. This explains why females experience much less hypertrophy than males. However, within each sex, there are large individual differences in the adaptation of muscles to training. Some males will respond more than others. Unfortunately it is difficult to predict who will respond and who will not. The same is true for females. As a rule the female who already shows signs of large muscle development is the one more likely to experience more hypertrophy from strength training than a less muscular female.

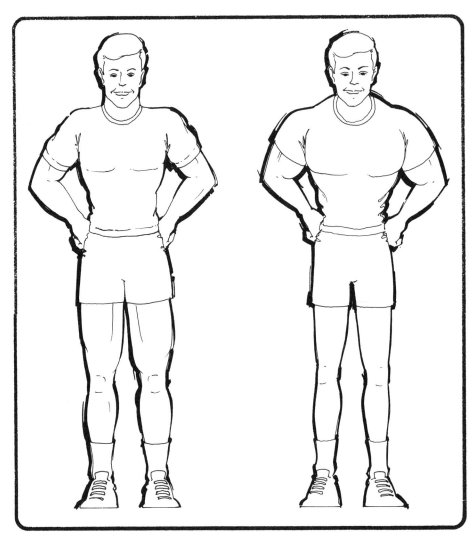

Figure 23: Muscle Building Programs Should be Designed to Symmetrically Develop the Whole Body Rather Than One Region Alone Such as the Upper Torso.

What Else?

Exercise helps control
obesity

Many persons of both sexes and all ages suffer from obesity (or excess body fat). Being overweight (or having more weight than average for one's height) is often but not always associated with obesity. Many football players are overweight but are not obese, for example. Measurements can be taken which can be used to predict whether one is overfat or not. Regular exercise done properly has been shown to be effective in treating obesity, and is also thought to help maintain a desired body weight and level of body fat (Figure 24).

How?

Prolonged aerobic
activities reduce
obesity

Included in the *Health Related Physical Fitness Test Manual* (AAHPERD, 1980) is a skinfold test for estimating the level of fatness in persons of both sexes and ages 5-18. Care must be taken in determining and interpreting such skinfold measures. Complete instructions are included in the test manual. A technical manual for this test has also been published recently (AAHPERD, 1984).

The recommended approach for reducing obesity is to combine a regular aerobic exercise program with a moderate diet. A moderate diet is defined as one which involves a total caloric intake of no fewer than 1200 kilocalories (kcal) per day, a caloric restriction of no more than 500-1000 kcal per day, and a maximum rate of weight loss of 1 kilogram (2.2 pounds) per week. The guidelines of the American College of Sports Medicine on proper and improper weight loss programs should be followed in undertaking any weight loss program (ACSM, 1984).

The most desirable exercises for preventing and treating obesity are ones in which the individual supports his/her body weight. Jogging is such an example. Many times, however, an obese person cannot jog effectively and so must resort to other exercise modes such as walking, cycling, or swimming. Longer and slower forms of exercise usually result in a greater total caloric expenditure. In general the most appropriate exercise procedure is one which causes the greatest total number of calories to be utilized and which brings the individual the most enjoyment. Prolonged aerobic activities are particularly beneficial for treating and preventing obesity. Evidence suggests that fat loss can be achieved in previously sedentary persons through regularly exercising a minimum of three times weekly for 20 minutes or longer.

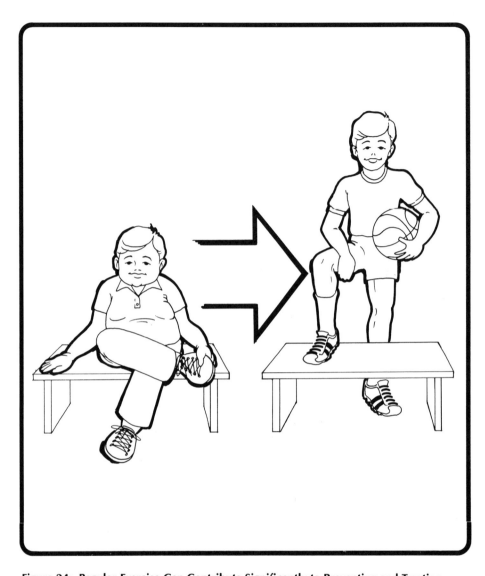

Figure 24: Regular Exercise Can Contribute Significantly to Preventing and Treating Obesity.

Why?

Inactivity more than food intake contributes to obesity

Evidence indicates that inactivity rather than excessive caloric intake may be a dominant cause of obesity. Obese individuals move less throughout the day but do not necessarily eat more. Habitual exercise of less than one hour does not necessarily cause an increase in appetite. Food intake may increase only to offset the increased caloric expenditure in some persons while in others intake may remain the same or even drop below the level of sedentary individuals. There is no evidence that regular exercise leads to the development of obesity by overstimulating the appetite.

The number of fat cells in humans increases until 16-18 years of age, thereafter remaining constant. In adulthood, gains in body fat come as a result of increases in fat cell size and not number. Obese persons usually have more fat cells than non-obese persons. Indirect evidence suggests that regular exercise during early life years when fat cells are being developed could help control obesity in adulthood.

Regular exercise is useful in treating obesity for a number of reasons. One relates to its effect on minimizing the reduction of resting energy expenditure which often occurs when an individual diets. Dieting (or reducing the caloric intake) is the most commonly practiced approach to treating obesity. By helping to keep the energy expenditure of the individual from dropping while on a diet, more fat is lost than otherwise would be the case. Literature on physical training programs indicates that while body weight may not change due to training, fat content is often reduced and lean tissue developed. Further analysis of the literature suggests that for a training program to cause a reduction in body fat the following minimum requirements must be met:

- the program must be conducted at least 3 times per week;
- it must last at least 20 minutes per day;
- it must be at a sufficient intensity and duration to expend approximately 300 kilocalories (kcal.) per exercise session. Note: a kcal. is the unit of caloric expenditure and is the same as "calorie" in lay terms.

As an example a 170 lb. male expends approximately 14.9 kcal. per minute when jogging at a pace of 9 minutes per mile (see Table 5). If he continues at that pace for 20 minutes, then the total caloric expenditure equals 298 kcal. [(14.9 kcal./min.) (20 min.) = 298 kcal.]. Jogging at a pace of 11.5 minutes per mile requires only 10.5 kcals. per minute. Therefore this person would need to jog for 28.5 minutes to achieve a total caloric expenditure of 300 kcal. per session at the slower pace [(300 cal.)/(10.5 kcal./min.) = 28.5 min.].

It should be noted in Table 5 that the number of kilocalories expended in an activity varies not only with the intensity or pace of the activity but also with body weight. The heavier the person the more kilocalories expended at a given pace. Females beyond puberty tend as a whole to weigh less than males. As a result they will need to engage in a given activity and at a given intensity for more time to achieve the goal of 300 kcal. per exercise session. Unfortunately the minimum requirements mentioned above emanate from data collected primarily on males. As more data are collected on females the recommended minimum daily caloric expenditure may be found to be less for females because of these differences in body weight.

There are several other reasons for including exercise in a program to reduce fat content. Weight loss by dieting alone causes loss of lean tissue and protein as well as fat whereas weight loss by exercise causes nearly all of the weight loss to come from fat. Regular exercise also contributes to the development of the muscular and cardiorespiratory systems as well as being useful in obesity treatment.

Aerobic exercise is of particular benefit since fat partially serves as a fuel for such work. Aerobic training promotes the development of enzymes involved in the breakdown of fat. This results in more fat being used as a fuel at a given level of work than before. Weight supported forms of exercise are preferable to others because more calories are spent in a specified period of time.

People often exercise to reduce fat in or around a specific location. Evidence suggests however that exercising a specific body part will not cause a reduction in localized fat deposits in that specific area.

Table 5: Energy Expenditure in Selected Activities (kcal/min)*

Activity	Kg 50 lb 110	59 130	68 150	77 170	86 190	95 209
Badminton	4.9	5.7	6.6	7.5	8.3	9.2
Basketball	6.9	8.1	9.4	10.6	11.9	13.1
Climbing Hills						
no load	6.1	7.1	8.2	9.3	10.4	11.5
with 10 kg load	7.0	8.3	9.5	10.8	12.0	13.3
Cycling						
5.5 mph	3.2	3.8	4.4	5.0	5.5	6.1
9.4 mph	5.0	5.9	6.8	7.7	8.6	9.5
Digging trenches	7.3	8.6	9.9	11.2	12.5	13.8
Forestry						
Ax chopping-fast	14.9	17.5	20.2	22.9	25.5	28.2
Ax chopping-slow	4.3	5.0	5.8	6.5	7.3	8.1
Gardening						
Mowing	5.6	6.6	7.6	8.6	9.6	10.6
Raking	2.7	3.2	3.7	4.2	4.6	5.1
Golf	4.3	5.0	5.8	6.5	7.3	8.1
Running						
Cross country (hills)	8.2	9.6	11.1	12.6	14.0	15.5
Level ground						
11.5 min/mi	6.8	8.0	9.2	10.5	11.7	12.9
9 min/mi	9.7	11.4	13.1	14.9	16.6	18.3
7 min/mi	12.2	13.9	15.6	17.4	19.1	20.8
Swimming						
Backstroke	8.5	10.0	11.5	13.0	14.5	16.1
Breaststroke	8.1	9.6	11.0	12.5	13.9	15.4
Crawl-fast	7.8	9.2	10.6	12.0	13.4	14.8
Crawl-slow	6.4	7.6	8.7	9.9	11.0	12.2
Tennis	5.5	6.4	7.4	8.4	9.4	10.4
Volleyball	2.5	3.0	3.4	3.9	4.3	4.8
Walking						
Comfortable pace	4.0	4.7	5.4	7.2	6.9	7.6
Sitting at ease	1.2	1.4	1.6	1.8	2.0	2.2
Writing	1.5	1.7	2.0	2.2	2.5	2.8
Lying at ease	1.1	1.3	1.5	1.7	1.9	2.1

*Adapted from Katch, F. & McArdle W. *Nutrition, Weight Control, and Exercise*. Boston: Houghton Mifflin Company, 1977, Appendix B: Energy Expenditure in Household, Recreational and Sports Activities (in Kcal/min).

coping

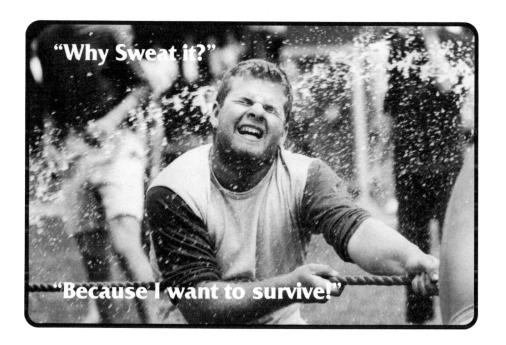

"Why Sweat it?"

"Because I want to survive!"

What Do You Have To Help Me?

In today's world "survival" can mean being free of disease. Many diseases are related to inadequate exercise. *Hypokinetic* degeneration is one such disease caused by insufficient movement. Handicapped persons are particularly susceptible to this disease because they are often not provided the means of fully using their bodies. Persons who suffer from hypokinetic degeneration can experience one or more of the following: bone and muscle atrophy; loss of flexibilty; cardiovascular degeneration; respiratory, bladder and bowel malfunction. Essentially all symptoms of hypokinetic degeneration can be reversed and even eliminated through proper exercise. Exercise has also proven to be of assistance in hastening the repair of fractured bones and in the recovery from injuries to muscles, tendons, and ligaments.

Lack of exercise is
involved in
hypokinetic
degeneration,
coronary heart
disease, and stroke

Coronary heart disease and *stroke* are two related diseases of great magnitude. Annually, close to 50 percent of the total deaths in the U.S. can be attributed to these diseases. Characteristics of people associated with premature susceptibility to these diseases are called risk factors. Lack of exercise is a secondary risk factor of significance in the development of both diseases. Two other risk factors, high blood pressure (hypertension) and obesity, are influenced by regular exercise. Exercise has been shown to have a small positive benefit to persons suffering from high blood pressure. Obesity has been successfully treated through a combination of exercise and diet.

How?

Adapted physical education programs are necessary

Regularly exercising all parts of the body in some comprehensive program is recommended for preventing and treating hypokinetic degeneration. Handicapped individuals are particularly in need of programs which focus on strength and range of motion. Such individuals also confront obesity and heart disease risk due to their inactivity. Adapted physical education programs are beneficial and of vital importance (Figure 25).

Large muscle rhythmic exercise for heart disease and stroke are recommended

Large muscle, rhythmic exercise is recommended for reducing the risk of coronary artery disease and stroke. Jogging, cross-country skiing, cycling, and swimming are all appropriate examples (Figure 26). The discussion of aerobic endurance training procedures in Chapter 1 outlines the recommended procedures in full.

Persons diagnosed as having coronary heart disease, stroke, or those who are in a higher risk category because of age or other known risk factors should avoid intensive small muscle exercises. Examples include push-ups and pull-ups (Figure 27). Isometric exercises should also be avoided because they demand a greater amount of blood to be pumped by the heart than at rest when the resistance to blood flow is increased. Rhythmic large muscle exercises also require more blood to be pumped by the heart than at rest, but the resistance to blood flow is reduced. The net effect of doing intensive small muscle exercises or any form of isometric exercise is that the heart muscle is forced into a very high workload presenting danger to anyone who has a potentially weak or diseased heart.

It is recommended that any inactive person over age 45 who is contemplating an exercise program should obtain a physical

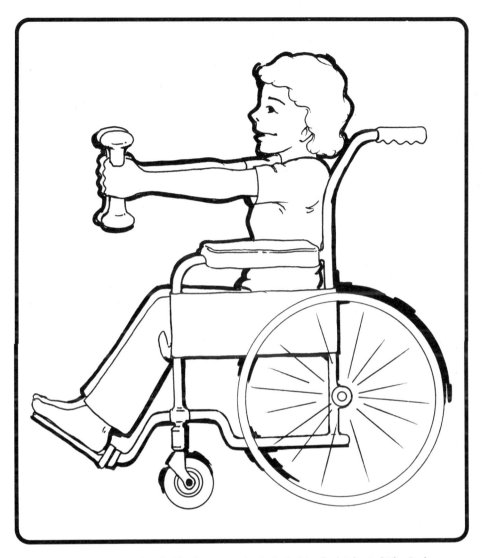

Figure 25: Handicapped Individuals are Particularly in Need of Adapted Physical Education Programs.

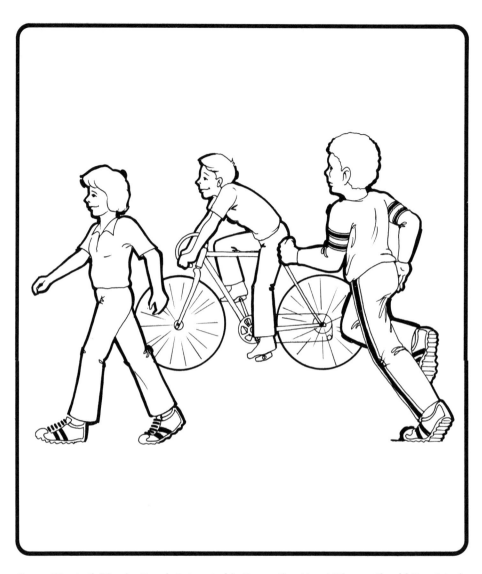

Figure 26: Activities for People Interested in Preventing Heart Disease Should Consist of Rhythmic Large Muscle Movements such as Cycling, Walking, and Jogging.

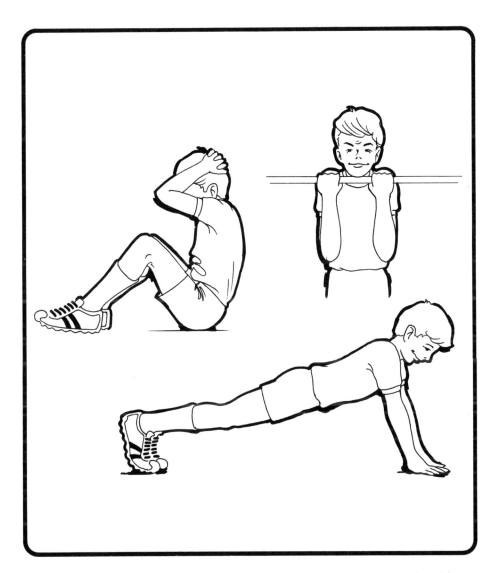

Figure 27: Isometric Exercise in General or Intensive Small Muscle Exercise Should be Avoided by People with Heart Conditions.

exam which evaluates the performance of the heart during such exercise. Such an exam is commonly referred to as an *exercise stress test*. Persons of any age who are at high risk should definitely receive such a stress test before beginning an exercise program. Anyone who has been diagnosed as having heart disease should exercise under the supervision of personnel who have been trained and/or certified by reputable institutions or organizations.

Why Does It Happen That Way?

Understanding the reasons why regular exercise prevents disease is very difficult because of the complexity of bodily processes and how diseases affect these processes. In Chapter 1 many beneficial changes from exercise in the muscular and circulatory systems were discussed. The relationship between obesity and exercise was discussed in Chapter 2. Some of the mechanisms not mentioned which relate exercise to the prevention and therapy of disease are presented in the following paragraphs.

If joints are not moved the connective tissue in ligaments, tendons, and muscle shortens, causing flexibility loss in the joint. Research has shown that connective tissue is strengthened by regular exercise; lack of exercise has the opposite effect.

Exercise helps to bind minerals into bones and connective tissue

Bone tissue is also affected by inactivity. Bones are constantly in a state of being modified and strengthened to meet the demands placed on them. Calcium and other minerals are deposited in stress areas. If the normal level of exercise is reduced, this strengthening process is interrupted and bones lose minerals making them weaker and more susceptible to fracture.

The relationship between lack of exercise and increased susceptibility to coronary artery disease and stroke has not been conclusively proven due to the complexity of the diseases and numerous contributing factors. In addition these diseases take many years to develop into a severe enough state to be diagnosed by present techniques. For these reasons research progress is slow. Although the role of inactivity is not yet proven there is enough indirect evidence for it to be listed as one of several secondary risk factors.

Many cardiologists feel that if the death rate from coronary artery disease and stroke is to be significantly lowered, something will have to be done to prevent rather than treat it once it appears. Since evidence suggests that these diseases may begin to develop in childhood it becomes evident that regular exercise habits need to be emphasized and established very early in life.

Exercise may help prevent heart disease and stroke

There are numerous reasons why exercise is thought to be related to the prevention of coronary heart disease and stroke. Research on rats has indicated that regular exercise promotes a larger arterial and capillary system feeding blood to the heart muscle. If this is also true in humans, more blood would flow to the heart muscle. Evidence suggests that regular exercise improves stroke volume by creating a greater contraction force. With a larger stroke volume the heart is able to pump blood through the body with fewer beats, thereby not having to work as hard.

Both high blood pressure and high blood fat levels are major risk factors in coronary heart disease and stroke. Exercise has been shown to be of some help in reducing high blood pressure. Other evidence suggests that exercise can favorably alter the composition of fats and cholesterol in the blood. As a result, the buildup of fatty deposits in the arterial walls may be slowed (Figure 28). The ability to break down clots may be increased through regular exercise. In all there are many potential explanations which could account for why regular exercise is thought to play a preventive role in the development of coronary artery disease and stroke (Figure 29).

Exercise is useful for cardiac rehabilitation

Exercise has proven to be of significant therapeutic benefit in the treatment of persons with known coronary artery disease for additional reasons. Clinical evidence suggests that such exercise programs contribute to a heightened physical work capacity in the person and less strain on the heart. This may occur even if the exercise does not improve the circulation to the heart muscle. The resulting effect on the individual is greater self-confidence and a heightened psychological outlook. The person is better equipped to regain a productive lifestyle. Tentative evidence suggests that all this results in a lowered rate of recurring problems and mortality.

What Else?

Surviving in emergencies

Living in the modern world requires the ability to survive in emergencies. Nobody can anticipate how or when a situation may arise requiring the ability to pull oneself up over a barrier, run fast, maintain a strong grip, or withstand a physical hardship. An adequate level of physical fitness (or adequate

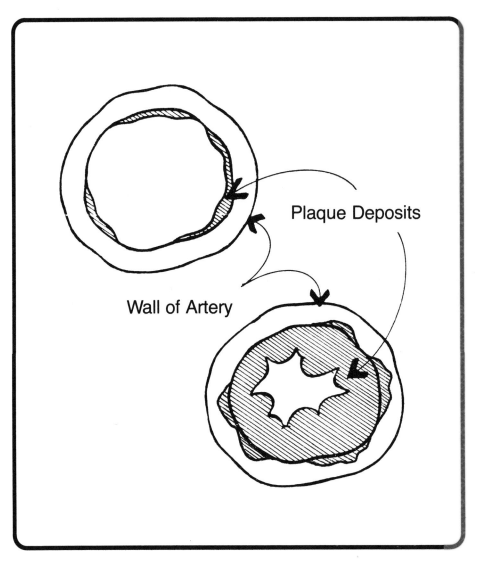

Figure 28: Regular Exercise May Slow the Building of Fatty Deposits on and Within the Walls of Arteries.

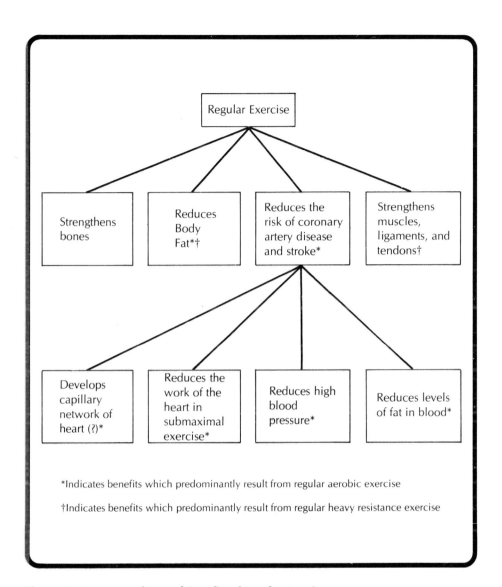

Regular Exercise

Strengthens bones

Reduces Body Fat*†

Reduces the risk of coronary artery disease and stroke*

Strengthens muscles, ligaments, and tendons†

Develops capillary network of heart (?)*

Reduces the work of the heart in submaximal exercise*

Reduces high blood pressure*

Reduces levels of fat in blood*

*Indicates benefits which predominantly result from regular aerobic exercise

†Indicates benefits which predominantly result from regular heavy resistance exercise

Figure 29: Summary of Several Benefits of Regular Exercise

strength, speed, and endurance) can make a crucial difference in such situations.

How?

Overall training for emergencies is desirable

Since one cannot predict if and when an emergency may arise, or what may be required for survival, a comprehensive approach to fitness is necessary.

To manage one's body weight, adequate strength in the upper body should be developed and maintained. Essentially one needs to train with near maximal weights or repeatedly exert near maximal force for strength development. Dynamic and isokinetic strength training techniques are appropriate methods (see Chapter 1). In addition, calisthenic exercises like pull-ups, push-ups, and dips can be satisfactorily employed where proper facilities for developing strength by these techniques are available.

Running speed can be improved through short term anaerobic training procedures. This involves running repeated intervals at near maximum speed (see Chapter 1).

Endurance implies either an ability to engage one muscle group in exercise over a long time period (muscular endurance) or the ability to engage the whole body in prolonged exercise (aerobic endurance). Muscular endurance training techniques involve repetitious exercise with a submaximal weight. Aerobic endurance training involves rhythmic large muscle exercise at least 15 minutes daily and 3 times per week at a pace which raises the heart rate to an adequate level. For the average young adult an adequate target heart rate to achieve in exercise ranges between 145-182 beats per minute. Persons who are particularly unfit when beginning may gain some benefit from exercises in which the heart rate is as low as 130 beats per minute. Both muscular and aerobic endurance training procedures were described in Chapter 1.

Circuit training

An alternative approach to overall fitness is *circuit training*. With this approach a series of individual exercises are tied into a circuit and then executed as quickly as possible. Often the exercises are located at different stations in a room. A great variety of individual exercises (stair running, push-ups, pull-ups, squat thrust, or flexibility exercises) may be used in devising a circuit. Weight lifting exercises are commonly used (Figure 30). Circuits can be varied according to individual needs or according to facility limitations. Persons can even organize their own circuits at home (Figure 31). A home based

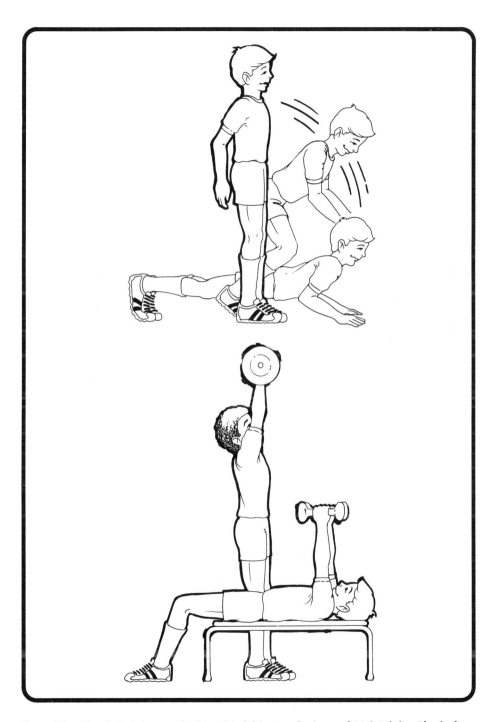

Figure 30: Circuit Training can be Very Useful in Developing and Maintaining Physical Fitness.

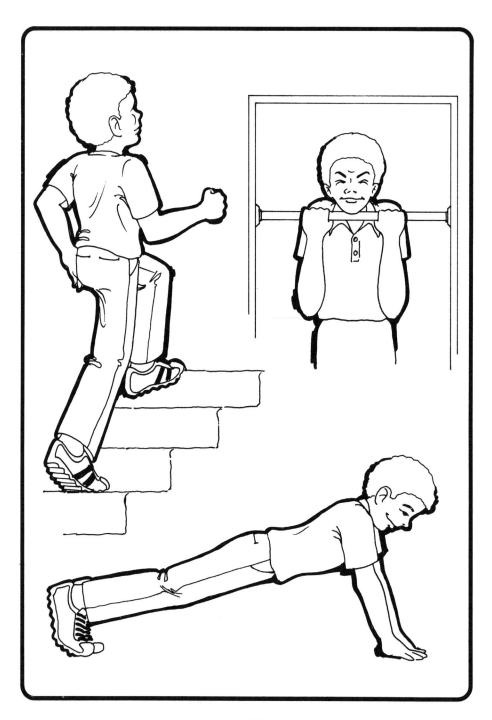

Figure 31: Possible Stations for a Home-Based Circuit Training Program.

circuit training program is of particular relevance for the handicapped individual. The overall individual benefit is the effect of each exercise on the specific body regions. In addition aerobic endurance can be increased to a modest degree from the continuous activity of going from station to station. This is particularly true if 30-45 seconds of large muscle activity (e.g. jogging in place, jumping rope) is interspersed between stations which focus on strength or muscle endurance.

health

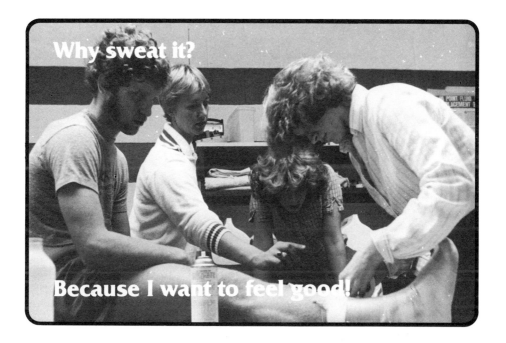

Why sweat it?

Because I want to feel good!

What Do You Have To Help Me?

It is not uncommon to experience muscular pain in the used body regions one or more days after heavy exercise. The term *muscle soreness* is used to described this pain. With proper techniques muscle soreness can be minimized or its severity reduced.

How?

Gradual increase in activity level lessens muscle soreness

Muscle soreness is maximized when the level of habitual activity is first raised as during the first week of an exercise program. The severity of the exercise also influences the de-

73

gree of muscle soreness a person will experience. Programs which cause a person to abruptly do much more exercise than she/he normally is accustomed to result in more muscle soreness than ones which slightly raise the level of activity. Therefore, it is advisable to use a gradual increase in activity level to prevent or minimize muscle soreness. Explosive, jerky, and maximal performances should be avoided. Use of thorough warm-up and cool down periods which involve stretching exercises are also recommended.

If and when muscle soreness develops, static stretching exercises of the sore regions have proven helpful in reducing pain. The technique simply involves holding the sore muscle in a stretched position for 15-30 seconds or longer (Figure 32). The exercise should be repeated several times a day if the pain is severe.

Why Does It Happen That Way?

Muscle soreness occurs from damage to muscle and/or connective tissue

The cause of muscle soreness is unclear, but recent evidence suggests that it is related to minor damage to the muscle cells and/or connective tissue. The effect of the damage is an altered fluid balance in the sore region for the next few days. This stimulates local nerve endings and causes pain. Evidence also has shown that soreness is more prevalent following heavy eccentric exercise (as in lowering a weight) than following heavy concentric exercise (as in raising a weight).

What Else?

Avoiding fatigue through fitness

Occasionally we are all called upon to physically use our bodies. A friend may need help lifting or carrying a load or somebody else may ask for assistance to move her/his household. In the spring it is not uncommon to see people cleaning up and digging in their gardens after months of indoor and relatively inactive living. Even the inactive person may find it difficult to refuse the invitation from a group of friends to take an afternoon bicycle ride on a sunny spring day. If an individual wishes the freedom to participate in a variety of such activities without being limited by premature fatigue, an adequate level of physical fitness is essential (Figure 33).

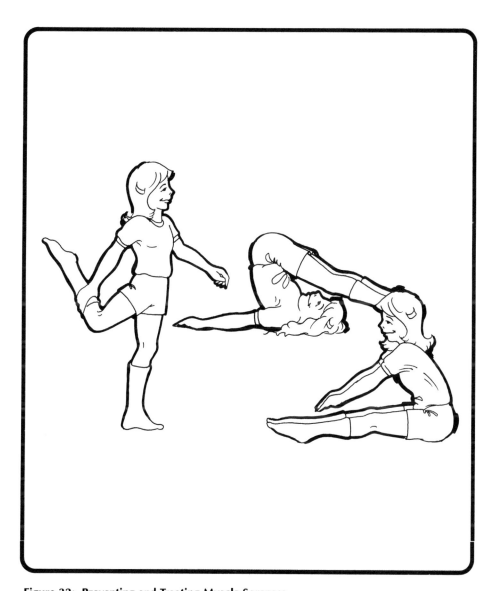

Figure 32: Preventing and Treating Muscle Soreness.
Static stretching exercises can minimize the amount of muscle soreness. Hold a stretched position for several seconds without bouncing.

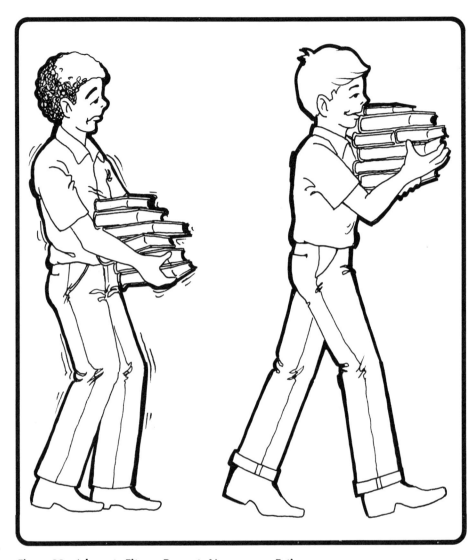

Figure 33: Adequate Fitness Prevents Unnecessary Fatigue.

How?

**Fatigue is minimized
through fitness**

Three fitness components seem to be of particular importance for "feeling good" while exercising.

Strength: Developing and maintaining an adequate level of muscular strength is important because strength appears to be involved to some degree in almost all performances. Persons with greater strength are likely to experience less fatigue than those with less strength. All regions of the body require adequate strength. Overemphasis on training only one body part does little to prepare the individual for the wide range of movements likely to be encountered while freely engaging in activity.

Two types of endurance, *muscular endurance* and *aerobic endurance,* appear to be of particular importance in minimizing premature fatigue from exercise. Muscular endurance refers to the ability of individual muscles to continue exercising for relatively long periods of time. Aerobic endurance refers to a similar ability of the whole body to persist in prolonged activity. If two otherwise equivalent persons who differed in levels of muscular and aerobic endurance were asked to work side by side on the same task, the one with the higher endurance would not only complete the task in less time but that person would experience more comfort during and afterwards. Training procedures to improve strength, muscle endurance, and aerobic endurance were described in Chapter 1.

One last word should be mentioned regarding feeling good while exercising. Persons who have excess body fat usually find themselves under greater strain while exercising at a given rate than those with low levels of body fat. This is because the fat acts as a heavy burden which must be borne along with the individual. Just as a heavy backpack slows down an exercising person by causing additional fatigue, so, too, does extra fat weight. The role of regular exercise in preventing and treating obesity is discussed in Chapter 2.

Why?

The explanation for a fit person's ability to exercise at a given level and feel better relates partly to the physiological and structural changes that occur from training. Any attempt to explain the phenomenon of feeling good (or not feeling good) while exercising should consider the causes and mechanisms of muscle fatigue.

Muscle fatigue is an exceedingly complex phenomenon which has no simple and entirely consistent explanation. Under some circumstances fatigue may result from a failure of the central nervous system to deliver impulses to the exercising muscles. Fatigue may also result when the junction between the nerve and the muscle does not perform adequately. The best explanation for muscle fatigue, however, is the failure of the muscle fibers to contract. This contraction failure may result from a variety of causes including depletion of energy sources, loss of substances required for contraction, and/or waste products accumulated during exercise.

In heavy exercise lasting less than 2-3 minutes, the needed ATP for muscle contraction is supplied primarily by anaerobic breakdown of creatine phosphate (CP) and muscle glycogen. A biproduct of the anaerobic breakdown of glycogen is lactic acid. Since neither CP nor glycogen levels are severely depleted in maximal exercise lasting less than 10 seconds (e.g. sprinting), it is thought that fatigue in such circumstances results from an inability to maintain the required level of ATP production. However, in heavy exercises which last longer than 10 seconds but less than approximately 2-3 minutes, fatigue is thought to result from the combined effects of CP depletion and lactic acid accumulation. It is not known whether lactic acid directly causes fatigue, whether fatigue results from the effect of lactic acid on lowering muscle pH, or whether both changes adversely affect the enzyme activity involved in anaerobic glycolysis.

An inadequate supply of oxygen to the muscle is also known to contribute to muscle fatigue. Such losses of oxygen supply are not uncommon in short-term, highly intensive levels of exercise, particularly if the exercise is isometric. The loss of oxygen supply to muscle is due to substantially reduced blood flow. Without adequate blood supply the delivery of oxygen and the elimination of waste from the muscle is disrupted.

When heavy exercise is continued for increasing periods beyond 2-3 minutes, the ability of a person's oxygen delivery systems to supply oxygen to the exercising muscles is of increasing importance in determining the level of work that can be sustained. However, anaerobic glycolysis appears to contribute to ATP production as well, particularly in performances that can only be sustained from 3-15 minutes. Fatigue in such circumstances is thought to be largely related to the build up of lactic acid.

There does not appear to be a single factor associated with

fatigue in heavy exercise lasting between 15 and 60 minutes. It has been suggested that fatigue in this case may result from a combination of a small increase in lactic acid, a modest decrease in muscle glycogen, and an increase in body temperature.

In prolonged exercise lasting 1-2 hours or more, fatigue appears strongly related to the depletion of muscle glycogen stores. In such circumstances a failure of temperature regulation resulting in heat exhaustion can also occur, particularly if one becomes dehydrated when exercising in the heat.

In light of the complexities of explaining muscle fatigue it is difficult to fully comprehend why training causes an improved response to a given level of exercise. The fact is that a trained person experiences less fatigue during and after the exercise when compared to an untrained individual of similar caliber working at the same work level. The net effect is that the trained individual "feels" better than the untrained one. Whether this arises out of a greater shortage of energy sources or fuel, a greater ability to tolerate the buildup of waste products or some combination of both, awaits further research. Psychological factors can also interact with the physiological factors, causing the trained individual to feel better than the untrained one.

What Else?

Low back pain can be lessened by strong abdominal muscles

Feeling good also concerns chronic low back pain considerations. It appears that many cases of low back pain can be prevented by maintaining good posture in the lower back region. The spine should be kept straight and should not be allowed to arch into the swayback position (Figure 34). Adequate flexibility of lower back and hamstring muscles coupled with adequate strength of the abdominal muscles is thought to contribute to the prevention of low back pain. Exercises which can be used to improve the strength and flexibility in these regions are described and illustrated in the *Health Related Physical Fitness Test Manual* (AAHPERD, 1980).

Physical activity enhances health and quality of life

Feeling good also relates to a person's overall health status. Whereas in Chapter 3 the role of exercise in preventing and treating disease was discussed, health implies more than freedom from disease. Health is a condition of the body characterized by vigor and vitality. Persons who partake in regular exercise usually enjoy an enhanced quality of life. Such ex-

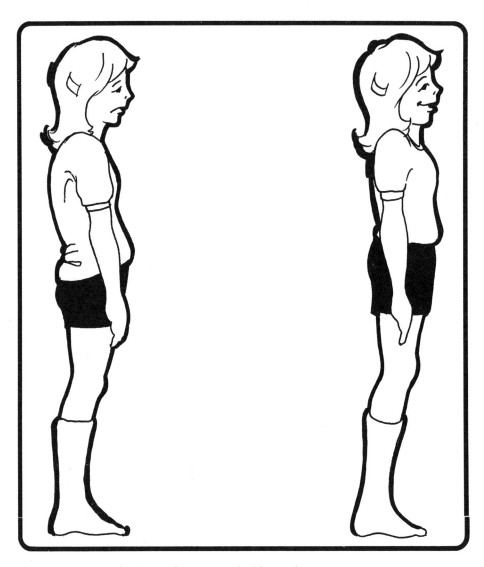

Figure 34: Low Back Pain can be Prevented with Good Posture.

ercise can come through regular training and/or by finding ways to incorporate exercise into daily living (Figure 35). Active people are able to more fully participate in life endeavors, responding with an enthusiasm and vigor that sometimes alienates their sedentary counterparts.

How?

**Regular exercise
should be tailored to
personal needs**

If an active lifestyle is to be achieved, it must be tailored to individual interests, talents, and means. While jogging and calisthenics may be effective for some, vigorous games or outdoor activities are more appropriate for others (Figure 36). It is unlikely that an individual will persist in activities that do not reap enjoyment. Therefore activities must be chosen which are compatible with individual interests and capabilities.

The approach into activity must be gradual for persons who have been sedentary for some time. Raising the activity level too rapidly can often result in injuries to tendons, ligaments, bones, and muscles. A gradual increase in activity status permits these structures to adapt and strengthen without ever exposing them to excessive strains that can contribute to injury. Through patience and slow progression the person desiring an enhanced quality of life through regular physical activity is more likely to feel good as progress is made. After approximately 4-5 months adequate structural and functional adaptations will have occurred to allow the individual to enter the maintenance phase of physical activity. This phase is characterized by a relative plateauing of the activity status of the individual, hopefully at a level which will allow the person to explore life to its fullest, with health and vigor, enthusiasm, and a sense of developing one's potential.

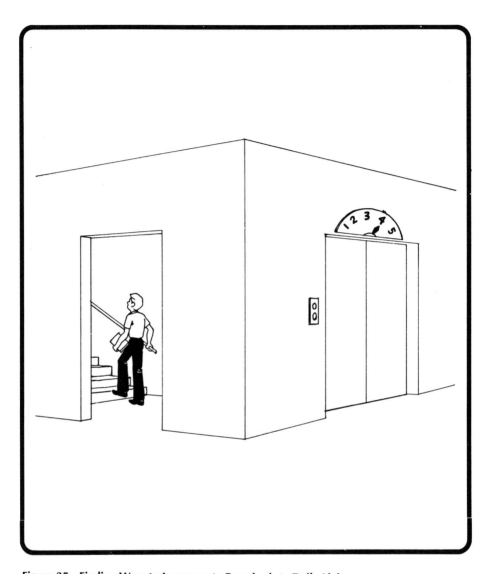

Figure 35: Finding Ways to Incorporate Exercise into Daily Living.

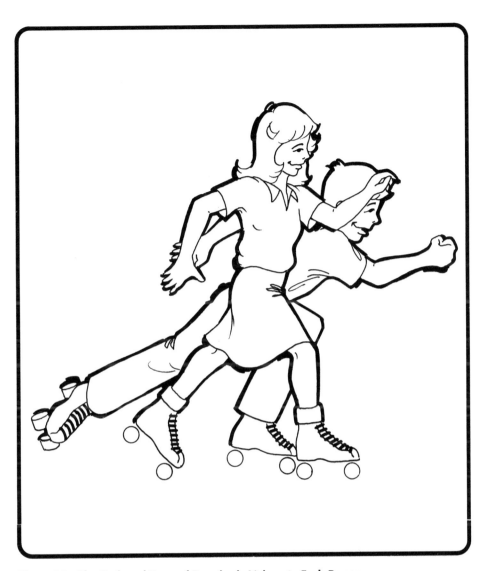

Figure 36: The Preferred Form of Exercise is Unique to Each Person.

CHAPTER FIVE

aesthetics/social/ psychological

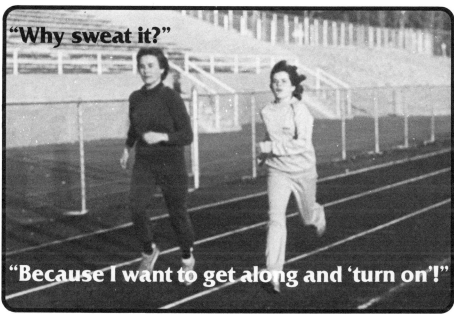

"Why sweat it?"

"Because I want to get along and 'turn on'!"

What Do You Have To Help Me?

Physical activity provides social benefits

By participating in activities which develop and maintain physical fitness a person will not only experience personal benefits but will also find that there will be plenty of opportunities to meet and interact with other people. For many, jogging with a friend is more pleasant than jogging alone. When people discover that they share the common interest of jogging, tennis, yoga, or other activities, a bond of common understanding is established between them. With the expanded interest in the racquet sports of tennis and racquetball and the necessary clubs and facilities to play these sports, many opportunities to interact with others arise (Figure 37). The same is true if one chooses to participate in the martial arts movements. Opportunities for social interaction have always existed in softball, basketball, or volleyball leagues. Op-

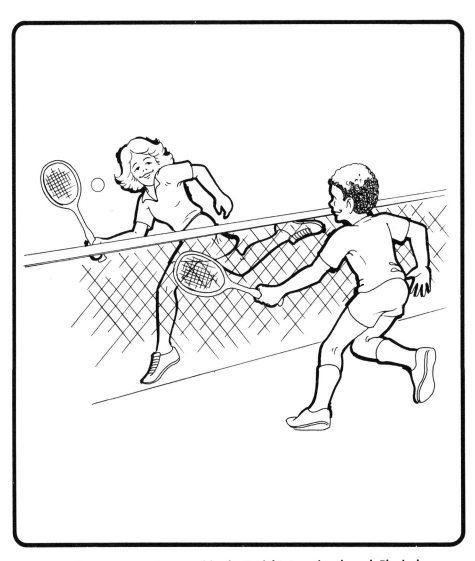

Figure 37: There are Many Opportunities for Social Interaction through Physical
Activity.

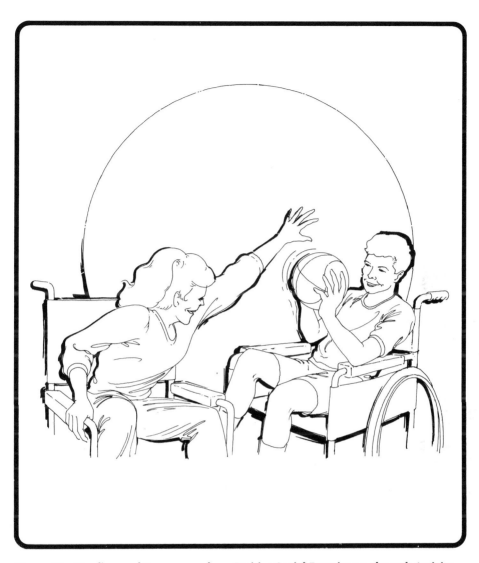

Figure 38: Handicapped Persons can have Positive Social Experiences through Activity.

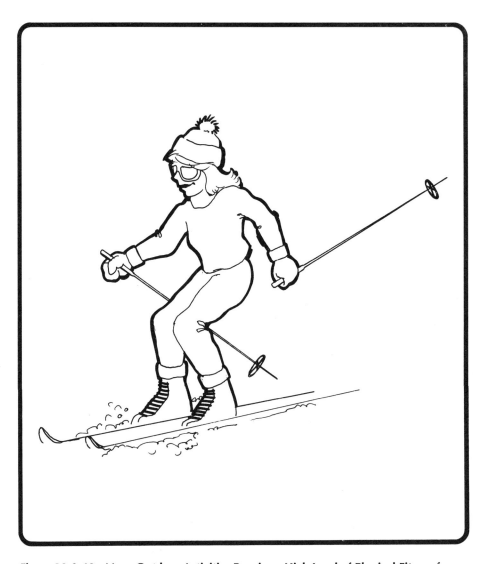

Figure 39 & 40: Many Outdoor Activities Require a High Level of Physical Fitness for Success and Safety.

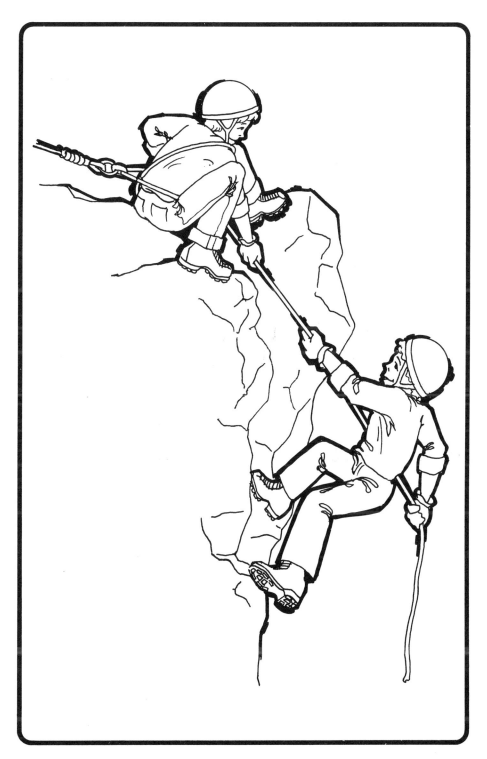

portunities for competition in swimming and track and field are ever growing in the number of varying ages of participants. Social interaction for handicapped individuals is becoming more available through sport and activity than in the past (Figure 38).

**Physical activity helps
to turn on**

For those who are "turned on" by the out-of-doors, adequate physical fitness is a necessity. The backpacker, the rock climber, the canoeist, or the skier, all must have the necessary fitness to do their respective activities as well as have the physical means to survive should an emergency arise (Figures 39 & 40).

A variety of self-enhancement movements are experiencing great popularity today. People are turning on by "getting into themselves" or by "listening to their bodies."A consistent theme running through all of the approaches to holistic self-development is the need to use and take care of the body through physical activity. Exercise is a part of life that our culture has progressively avoided. As people find themselves unfulfilled in their current lifestyles they often search for means of filling some of the voids. Many discover that much of this searching can be resolved by adopting a lifestyle which strives toward achieving a balance. Part of that balance inevitably includes physical activity (Figure 41).

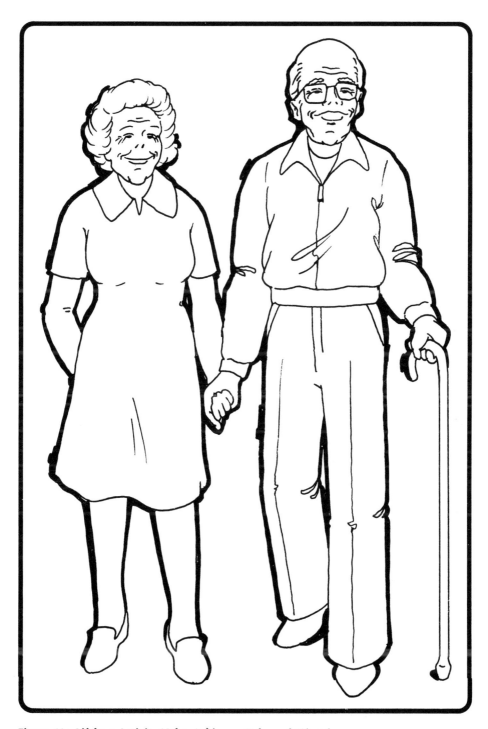

Figure 41: Lifelong Activity Helps Achieve a Balanced Lifestyle.

Selected References

AAHPERD. (1980). *Health related physical fitness: Test manual*. Reston, VA.

American College of Sports Medicine position statement on prevention of thermal injuries during distance running. (October, 1984). *Medicine and Science in Sports and Exercise, 16,* ix-xiv.

American College of Sports Medicine position statement on proper and improper weight loss programs. (1983). *Medicine and Science in Sport and Exercise, 15*(1), ix-xiii.

American College of Sports Medicine position statement on the use of anabolic-androgenic steroids in sports. (July, 1984). *Sports Medicine Bulletin.*

American College of Sports Medicine position statement on the recommended quantity and quality of exercise for developing and maintaining fitness in healthy adults. (1978). *Medicine and Science in Sports, 10*(3), vii-ix.

Astrand, P.O. and Rodahl, K. (1986). *Textbook of work physiology, 3rd ed.* New York: McGraw Hill.

Brooks, G.A. & Fahey, T.D. (1984). *Exercise physiology: Human bioenergetics and its applications*. New York: John Wiley and Sons.

deVries, H.A. (1986). *Physiology of exercise, 4th ed.* Dubuque, IA: Wm. C. Brown.

Falls, H.B., Jackson, A.S., Lohman, T., Nelson, J., Pate, R.R., Plowman, S., Safrit, M.J. & Ciszek, R.A. (1984). *Technical manual: Health related physical fitness*. Reston, VA: AAHPERD.

Fox, E.L. (1984). *Sports physiology, 2nd ed.*. Philadelphia: W.B. Saunders.

Fox, E.L. and Mathews, D.K. (1981). *The physiological basis of physical education and athletics, 3rd ed.* Philadelphia: Saunders College Publishing.

Hunsicker, P. & Reiff, G.G. (1976). *AAHPERD youth fitness test manual*. Reston, VA.

Katch, F.I. & McArdle, W.D. (1983). *Nutrition, weight control and exercise, 2nd ed.* Philadelphia: Lea and Febiger.

Lamb, D.R. (1984). *Physiology of exercise, 2nd ed.* New York: MacMillan Publishing Co.

McArdle, W.D., Katch, F.I., & Katch, V.L. (1986). *Exercise physiology, 2nd ed.* Philadelphia: Lea and Febiger.

National children and youth fitness study (January, 1985). *JOPERD, 56*(1), 44-90.

Noble, B.J. (1986). *Physiology of exercise and sport*. St. Louis: Times Mirror/Mosby College Publishing.

Pollock, M.L., Wilmore, J.H., & Fox III, S.M. (1984). *Exercise in health and disease*. Philadelphia: W.B. Saunders.

Sharkey, B.J. (1984). *Physiology of fitness, 2nd ed.* Champaign, IL: Human Kinetics Publishers.

Stull, G.A. (Ed.). (1980). *Encyclopedia of physical education, fitness and sports: Training, environment, nutrition and fitness*. Salt Lake City: Brighton Publ. Co.

Wilmore, J.H. (1982). *Training for sport and activity: The physiological basis of the conditioning process, 2nd ed.* Boston: Allyn and Bacon, Inc.

CARROLL COLLEGE LIBRARY